FOOD AND BEVERAGE CONSUMPTION AND HEALTH

GINGER

ANTIOXIDANT PROPERTIES, FUNCTIONS AND MEDICINAL BENEFITS

FOOD AND BEVERAGE CONSUMPTION AND HEALTH

Additional books in this series can be found on Nova's website under the Series tab.

Additional e-books in this series can be found on Nova's website under the e-book tab.

FOOD AND BEVERAGE CONSUMPTION AND HEALTH

GINGER

ANTIOXIDANT PROPERTIES, FUNCTIONS AND MEDICINAL BENEFITS

JANINE L. PERRY
EDITOR

nova publishers
New York

NOTICE TO THE READER

Library of Congress Cataloging-in-Publication Data

ISBN: 978-1-63482-020-2
Library of Congress Control Number: 2015930586

Published by Nova Science Publishers, Inc. † New York

CONTENTS

PREFACE

This book discusses all of the properties, as well as its functions and the medicinal benefits of ginger.

Chapter 1 - *Zingiber officinale* Roscoe (ginger) has been used in popular medicine since ancient times, being explored for its effects anti-inflammatory, antiemetic, anti-microbial and several other properties by both common folk and scientific community. Apart from its well-known folklore uses, there are several more studies that can be found in scientific research which describe many other capabilities of this plant. Also, several investigations have associated ginger with medicinal benefits, as antioxidant, anti-inflammatory and analgesic, antiemetic, anti-diarrheal, anti-ulcer, anti-cancer, anti-cholinesterasic, anti-bacterial, anti-fungal, anti-parasitary and preventing intoxications. So this chapter was prepared with the aim to contribute to the understanding of ginger, its general characteristics, physicochemical properties, pharmacological and toxicological properties as well as elucidating biochemical mechanisms whenever possible. Several beneficial and applicable effects of ginger have already been vastly studied and documented, such as the anti-inflammatory properties. Recent researches demonstrate that ginger possesses still other applications, and it could be useful in the treatment cardiovascular diseases and other metabolic problems. It is important to state that the antioxidant activity of ginger's phenolics is the main property responsible for the majority of the other effects described in this review. Studies published in the few past decades to more recent years will be presented.

Chapter 2 - The use of medicinal plants for developing new medications with therapeutic potential deservedly stands out in research. Numerous medicinal species have been reported in the literature, with promising possibilities of discovery of new drugs and also other products, with different potential uses. Ginger (*Zingiber officinale* Roscoe 1807) is of particular interest among these species, since it has been known for millennia and has been widely used by the population, mostly in cookery. Research on the chemical composition of ginger has indicated that it has important biological activity such as antimicrobial and antioxidant action, among other forms of activity. Because of these chemical characteristics, ginger has wide-ranging pharmacological use, with action on metabolism activity and use in treating diseases such as obesity (which is a risk factor for cardiovascular diseases), some types of cancer, psychological disorders and diabetes, among others. Studies have shown the worryingly negative aspects of obesity with regard to the population's health. Thus, adding foods that can enhance metabolic activity, as is the case with ginger, has a direct influence on excessive food intake and constitutes a promising strategy. In addition to characteristics relating to pharmacology, other potential uses broaden the functionality of ginger, such as the fact that this species is considered to be a potential insecticide. Plant extracts from ginger have been used in several types of insect pest control. Moreover, results from research have indicated that ginger can be multifunctional for agriculture, with contributions towards management and control of several food production chains, which broadens the diversity of new products used in agriculture, with the aim of integrated management for agricultural production, thus ensuring food quality. This chapter addresses some interesting aspects of research on the use of ginger for the treating various illnesses and also indicates its potential use in controlling and managing sustainable agricultural production. Ginger is a multifunctional medicinal species, with diverse actions and wide-ranging use for development of new products.

Chapter 3 - The rhizome, stem and leaves of ginger (*Zingiber officinale*) exhibit antioxidant activity. However, the bulk of studies was done using the rhizome extract and some were performed using the essential oil. Compounds have been isolated and chemically characterized from ginger. The anti-diabetic, neuroprotective, gastroprotective, nephroprotective, and cardio-protective actions of ginger are related to its antioxidant activity. Ginger has a beneficial effect on male reproduction in rodents and broiler chickens. It ameliorates the toxicity of insecticides. These actions may also be related to its antioxidant activity.

Chapter 4 - Ginger displays protective effects on Alzheimer's disease. It brings about attenuation of neuroinflammation and cognitive deficits. It exhibits anti-inflammatory, anticancer, antihypercholesterolemic, hepato-protective, anti-rheumatoid arthritis, antinociceptive, anti-viral, antischistosomal and insecticidal activities. It inhibits bacterial biofilm formation. It prevents nausea and vomiting, and exerts a protective effect on the metabolic syndrome-associated kidney injury. It decreases the severity of symptoms of premenstrual syndrome.

Chapter 5 - Ginger is a world known food plant which is equally reputed for its food flavoring and medicinal properties. 6-Gingerol is the major phenolic plant secondary metabolite present in the rhizome of ginger. This chapter reports chemical structure, biosynthesis, analytical methods and pharmacology as well as most recent research findings on potential cardiovascular health benefits of 6-gingerol. Qualitative and quantitative analytical techniques for the analysis of 6-gingerol and for the determination of the metabolism and bioavailability of 6-gingerol are discussed. Analytical techniques used for 6-gingerol that are described in this chapter are thin-layer chromatography (TLC), high-performance liquid chromatography (HPLC) combined with various detectors, and nuclear magnetic resonance (NMR) spectroscopy. The potential cardiovascular health effects of 6-gingerol include, anti-atherosclerotic, anti-platelet aggregation and antihypertensive effects as well as fibrinolytic activity.

Chapter 6 - In this study, a gas chromatography–mass spectrometry method in EI mode is developed for the analysis of dried Korean ginger. Hydro distillation–headspace solvent microextraction with polar and non-polar solvents is used. Forty-nine compounds are separated and identified. Some of the ginger compounds partially or completely were thermally decomposed. Some of these decomposition products likely produced when ginger is used in cooking at high temperatures and subsequently eaten. The major compounds in the rhizome identified are α-zingiberene, curcumene, camphene, β-phellandrene, (E)-citral, α-farnesene, β-bisabolene, β-sesquiphellandrene, zingerone, and [6]-gingerol. This method will be useful for rapid screening purpose of plant samples for finding of high quality ginger under the plant breeding program, genotypes assessment, and also export quality of ginger species.

Chapter 7 - Researchers have for many decades been trying to develop new broad-spectrum antibiotics against the infectious diseases caused by bacteria. Prolonged usage of these broad-spectrum antibiotics has led to the emergence of drug resistance. Resistance to antimicrobial agents has become an increasingly important and pressing global problem. There is a tremendous need for novel antimicrobial agents from different sources.

Plants used in traditional medicine are still understudied, particularly in clinical microbiology. So seeking for the *in vitro* antimicrobial activity of natural compounds such as polyphenols from ethnomedicinal plants on pathogenic bacteria is a new challenge.

Therefore, the authors investigated the possibility of the plants having the capacity to confront these bacteria.

In: Ginger
Editor: Janine L. Perry

ISBN: 978-1-63482-020-2

Chapter 1

ZINGIBER OFFICINALE ROSCOE, A PLANT OF MULTIPLE USES: A REVIEW OF PAST AND RECENT RESEARCH

Gustavo Henrique Oliveira da Rocha, Simone Aparecida Galerani Mossini and Miguel Machinski Junior*

Laboratory of Toxicology, Department of Basic Health Sciences
State University of Maringa, Maringa, Brazil

ABSTRACT

Zingiber officinale Roscoe (ginger) has been used in popular medicine since ancient times, being explored for its effects anti-inflammatory, antiemetic, anti-microbial and several other properties by both common folk and scientific community. Apart from its well-known folklore uses, there are several more studies that can be found in scientific research which describe many other capabilities of this plant. Also, several investigations have associated ginger with medicinal benefits, as antioxidant, anti-inflammatory and analgesic, antiemetic, anti-diarrheal, anti-ulcer, anti-cancer, anti-cholinesterasic, anti-bacterial, anti-fungal, anti-parasitary and preventing intoxications. So this chapter was prepared with the aim to contribute to the understanding of ginger, its general

*Corresponding author: Miguel Machinski Junior. Laboratory of Toxicology, Department of Basic Health Sciences, State University of Maringa, Maringa, 87020-900, Brazil. E-mail: machinski.jr@gmail.com or mmjunior@uem.br.

characteristics, physicochemical properties, pharmacological and toxicological properties as well as elucidating biochemical mechanisms whenever possible. Several beneficial and applicable effects of ginger have already been vastly studied and documented, such as the anti-inflammatory properties. Recent researches demonstrate that ginger possesses still other applications, and it could be useful in the treatment cardiovascular diseases and other metabolic problems. It is important to state that the antioxidant activity of ginger's phenolics is the main property responsible for the majority of the other effects described in this review. Studies published in the few past decades to more recent years will be presented.

Keywords: Ginger, biological properties, review

INTRODUCTION

Zingiber officinale Roscoe, known popularly as ginger, is a plant belonging to the Zingiberaceae family. Although its most popular use is as a spice, ginger has been used widely in Asian countries for medicinal purposes for centuries. Some of ginger's common uses include: antiemetic, cardiotonic, anti-inflammatory, hypoglycemic, antibacterial, anti-tumor, antifungal and antioxidant. More accurately, the rhizome is the main part used for all of these effects [1].

Increasing search for natural substances with pharmacological actions has given researchers wide field for studies. Population tends to have more acceptances towards natural products, such as herbs and roots.

However, ginger usage must have a cautious approach: even possessing lots of therapeutic uses, ginger can also cause toxic reactions if misused [2], as expected from any other plant.

There are several studies published in the last years that verify ginger`s pharmacological properties, as well as its major components that provide such effects. Literature already contains some reviews concerning ginger [1,3,4], as well as specific reviews that evaluate some of its effects on human health, such as its effects on the cardiovascular system [5], its antiemetic properties [6,7], and its anti-cancer properties [8].

This review has as its objective to summarize the uses of ginger and its pharmacological properties present in the scientific literature, including both older and more recent research.

CHEMISTRY

The great number of uses ginger has is due to the large number of chemical compounds it possesses. Although there are several chemical components, most of them can be identified as phenolic structures, such as the gingerols, which are responsible for antioxidant properties [9, 10]. Flavonoids are also included among ginger's chemical components [11].

Volatile terpenoids can also be found, responsible for the characteristic odor of ginger [12].

It is important to note that there aren't academic papers where the authors fully agree on the main chemical components found in ginger's rhizome. This is expected, since compounds present in the rhizome tend to vary greatly according to the precedence of the rhizome, growth and storage conditions, extraction methods and identification methods used.

The most common methods to obtain the chemical components include extraction with solvents [9, 13, 14] and, in some cases, the use of supercritical fluid, such as carbon dioxide – CO_2 [9, 10].

Use of different co-solvents have already been studied, and although different possibilities exist, like ethanol, isopropyl alcohol, acetone, hexane and petroleum ether, each results in ginger extracts with different components [9,14]. Harvest season, drying and storage manner cause alterations in the composition of ginger extracts [15]. Photosynthesis interferes with the production of primary and secondary metabolites, therefore the influence of light and CO_2 can influence the pathways of major chemical components [16, 17]. The different forms of rhizome processing interfere in its composition, as it can be sliced or triturated before extraction [18].

Finally, in the majority of studies, ginger's chemicals are usually analyzed through gas spectrometry coupled to mass spectrometry [13-15], which has been proven a reliable method of analysis of not only ginger extracts, but extracts from other plants as well.

Figure 1 shows the major components of ginger oil and ginger extracts: zingiberene, 6-gingerol and shogaols [9, 10, 15].

As it would be expected, most studies about ginger pharmacological properties involve particularly these compounds.

Of course, these are only the main chemicals, but there is an infinity of other compounds that can be found in ginger in smaller amounts: geranial, neral, geraniol, eucalyptol, canfen, geranyl acetate, ß-bisabolen, ß-felandren, camphor, myrcene, and many others [11, 13, 15].

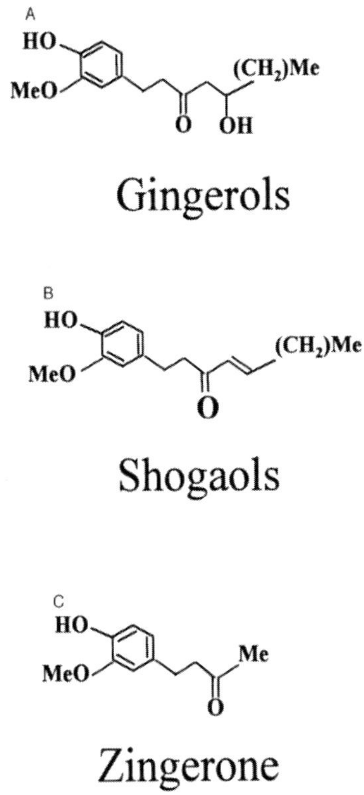

Figure 1. Main chemical compounds found in ginger oil/extracts. A: gingerol basic structure; B: shogaol basic structure; C: zingerone.

PHARMACOLOGICAL PROPERTIES

Antioxidant Property

All phenolic components, from geraniols to shogaols, are responsible to some extension for the antioxidant effects of ginger's rhizome. Researchers had used various methods to show this effect, and the most common methods employed are the DPPH (20-diphenyl-1-picrylhydrazyl), thiobarbituric acid and ferric thiocyanate radical scavenging assays. The antioxidant potential of ginger in these studies is comparable to common synthetic antioxidants, such as BHT (butyl hidroxylated toluene), even surpassing them in some studies [11, 13, 19].

Many intoxications and diseases are associated with free oxygen radicals. As ginger helps nullifying them, it is no surprise that many problems related to free radicals can be attenuated by ginger's extract. For example, studies demonstrated that cisplatin induces nephropathy by depleting the antioxidant renal systems by lowering reduced glutathione levels. Ginger extracts can scavenge the free radicals generated by cisplatin, maintaining the glutathione levels tolerable and preventing renal damage [20]. Acetaminophen induces hepatotoxicity by the same way, ginger extracts prevent the depletion of reduced glutathione and improve the antioxidant status of the liver, keeping the damage to a minimum [21]. In gastric ulcer models, the gastrointestinal damage causes increase in the levels of enzymes xanthine oxidase and myeloperoxidase, administration of ginger extracts can attenuate the increase in enzyme activity caused by oxidative distress generated by neutrophils and lipid peroxidation [22]. Generation of free radicals caused in arthritis conditions also increases superoxide dismutase and catalase levels and decreases the concentration of reduced gluthatione, ginger extracts are capable of stabilizing the activity of such enzymes and also of restoring the reduced glutathione levels [23].

Most studies found in the literature were performed with ginger extracts, but some show research done with isolated ginger compounds, in order to find a specific chemical with the most antioxidant capability. Several components have been obtained as derivates from zingiberene, one major ginger component. Studies with such derivates elucidated that the number and position of hydroxyl groups attached to the main aromatic structure are critical to the antioxidant activity of zingiberene. Since zingiberene is one of the phenolics present in ginger, it is suggested that other phenolics should work the same way [24]. Another substance, 6-gingerol, is a compound frequently studied, it is a potent inhibitor of oxidation caused by nitric oxide and its derivates, and it also prevents DNA damage caused by the formation of peroxynitrite.

In HepG2 cells subjected to radiation at LD50 doses, pre-treatments with 6-gingerol are capable of reducing cell death and regulating the activity of enzymes catalase and superoxide dismutase. Since nitric oxide synthesis and formation of radicals rely on reactions involving oxygen and superoxides, and that the activity of the enzymes superoxide dismutase and catalase are related directly to the intensity of oxidative distress, the activities of 6-gingerol reinforce the fact that ginger's polyphenols are strong antioxidants [25, 26].

Although the majority of studies performed with ginger made use only of the rhizomes, leaves and stem also have radical scavenging properties.

Even if the exact components and their proportions vary depending on the part of the plant, polyphenols can always be encountered in the whole plant, and not only in the rhizome. Rhizome and leaves have almost the same antioxidant capacity. The stem, however, exhibits only half the antioxidant potential shown by the other plant parts [11].

Anti-Inflammatory and Analgesic Properties

One of ginger's most common uses is as an analgesic, due to its anti-inflammatory properties. It is known that the inflammatory response that generates pain is mediated by a lot of factors, and ginger is capable of interfering with the inflammatory response through many of these factors. Scientific literature even has reviews dedicated to this matter alone [27].

Anti-inflammatory action of ginger comes from the inhibition of inflammatory prostaglandins. This happens because most of ginger's phenolic compounds, mainly 6-gingerol, are capable of inhibiting COX-2, thus preventing inflammatory prostaglandins, like PGE2, from being synthesized; 5-LIPOX is also inhibited, preventing leukotriene synthesis. A study demonstrated that not only 6-gingerol, but also 10-gingerol, 12-gingerol, 8-shogaol, 10-shogaol, 6-gingerdione, 8-gingerdione, 10-gingerdione, 6-paradol and 8-paradol are all capable of inhibiting COX-2; 10-gingerol, 8-shogaol and 10-shogaol are also receptor-specific, capable of inhibiting COX-2 without interacting with COX-1. Even though this inhibition is not very strong, it certainly demonstrates that ginger's chemicals show potential as base structures for future development of anti-inflammatory drugs [28].

Studies performed with rodents which employed induced skin edema, acetic acid induced writhing, induced arthirtis and hot-plate models of induced inflammation, demonstrated preeminent value of ginger anti-inflammatory properties. In these studies, ginger-treated animals developed less skin edema, took more time to writhe and lick the forepaws, and paws exhibited less redness and swelling when compared to non-treated animals [23, 29-32]. In one of these studies, the prevention of inflammation effects caused by adjuvant arthritis was shown to be directly linked to COX-2 inhibition by ginger [32].

Another study using the rat skin edema model again demonstrated that inflammation can be attenuated by a ginger extract, however, the authors induced the inflammatory process for more than 4 hours, and at this point, no longer is the inflammation modulated by eicosanoids. Instead, it is regulated by serotonin, released by degranulation of mast cells. This study suggests that ginger extracts not only inhibited prostaglandin synthesis, but could as well act as an antagonist of serotonin, being able to prevent inflammation for a long time through this mechanism [33]. Ginger also reduces C-reactive protein levels, which also contributes to preventing inflammation [34].

In vitro studies are also described in the literature; they demonstrate that ginger can attenuate the inflammatory response through other pathways as well. Ginger extracts successfully inhibit PGE2 production by U937 lineage cells; again, this happens because ginger compounds inhibit COX-2. However, the inhibition may happen at more than one site, as such compounds can inhibit not only the enzyme COX-2 itself, but they can also interfere with COX-2 mRNA stability [35]. NF-kappaB is a transcription factor crucial for initiation of inflammatory cytokines production such as TNF- α, IL-1 and IL-6, as well as nitric oxide. The production of these cytokines induced by lipid peroxidation in BV-2 microglial cells and by Il-1ß treatment in HuH-7 hepatic cells was inhibited by ginger extracts, which suggests that ginger compounds interfere with these pathways, directly modulating the gene expression for these cytokines [36, 37]. Ginger can also reduce T lymphocytes proliferation and differentiation *in vitro*, and since T lymphocytes are also involved in the cytokines pathways for inflammation, this is also a valid mechanism for ginger's anti-inflammatory properties [38].

Studied as the most preeminent phenolic compound active in ginger extracts, 6-gingerol alone is capable of reducing carragenin-induced paw edema in mice, as well as reducing mice writhing caused by acetic acid [39]. Such compound inhibits the production of pro-inflammatory cytokines such as IL-1, IL-12 and TNF-α in macrophages *in vitro*, probably acting through the NF-kappaB pathway. Besides, 6-gingerol acts as an antioxidant, scavenging the free radicals generated in distress conditions [40].

In another study, it is reported that ginger extracts attenuate allergic inflammation induced by ovoalbumin in mice lungs. Production of inflammatory cytokines in allergic reactions such as IL-4 and IL-5 which induces Th-2 response is greatly decreased. The recruitment of macrophages, neutrophilis and eosinophilis is also inhibited. Posterior tests using 6-gingerol, 10-gingerol and 6-shogaol gave very similar results concerning the suppression of allergic inflammatory reaction. This demonstrated that ginger has also possibilities in allergy treatment [41, 42].

A very throughout study demonstrated that another compound found in ginger, 1-dehydro-[10]-gingerdione, is capable of preventing inflammatory response of macrophages induced with LPS through several mechanisms that culminate in the prevention of NF-kappaB gene expression, which then reduces release of several other inflammatory cytokines [43].

There are also clinical trials that evaluated ginger anti-inflammatory properties. A study with patients with osteoarthritis demonstrated that subjects treated with ibuprofen (a classical non-steroidal COX-2 inhibitor) and ginger extract had their pain alleviated, with no significant difference between the drug and the extract [44]. Other study related to osteoarthritis also shows that ginger ameliorated pain in a long-run treatment, as the patients related pain decrease after 3 months of ginger administration [45]. In a study performed with young women suffering from dysmenorrhea, ginger capacity in reducing pain is comparable to ibuprofen and mefenamic acid [46]. Ginger was also capable of reducing pain generated by exercise; in another study, after eccentric exercise, arm pain was not so strong if ginger was administered to the subjects during the test. However, as PGE2 levels remain the same during exercise, ginger is supposed to alleviate pain through another unclear ways that do not involve prostaglandins [47].

Antiemetic Property

Ginger has also been vastly used as an antiemetic in common folk medicine. As well as the anti-inflammatory properties, this is already a vastly studied topic. There are reviews in the literature dedicated to this topic alone [6,7]. Most of the research done upon this matter dates back to before year 2000, but there are recent studies that further expand the subject.

Ginger is able to reduce motion sickness at the same extension as the anti-histamine dimenhydrinate. Both delay the time it takes to vomiting and nausea to happen in human subjects, but eventually, the neural component related to emesis surpasses the gastric component and vomiting is inevitable. This suggested that ginger probably acts in the gastrointestinal system, and not in the central nervous system [48]. Another study expands the motion sickness topic; ginger prevents gastric dysrhythmias, which precedes emesis, and does not only delay vomiting, but also shortens its recovery. Also, ginger prevents the release of vasopressin, which is one of the factors that contribute to nausea [49]. In dogs, ginger prevents cisplatin induced emesis. The authors suggested that 6-gingerol antagonizes serotoninergic receptors like 5-HT_3 and acts as an antioxidant, scavenging free radicals and preventing gastric distress [50].

Emesis can be caused due to radiation exposure, and ginger extracts attenuate that as well. More precisely, radiation exposure induces taste aversion which leads to emesis depending of what is eaten; treatment of rats exposed to radiation with ginger and anti-emetic drugs such as dexamethasone and ondansteron resulted in similar effects in returning the animals to normal dietary conditions. Again, this probably occurs due to 5-HT_3 inhibition and radical scavenging in the stomach [51].

Some compounds found in ginger were isolated and tested for receptor interaction, and it was demonstrated that chemicals 6-gingerol, 8-gingerol, 10-gingerol and 6-shogaol are capable of a slight antagonistic effect on cholinergic M_3 and serotoninergic 5-HT_5 receptors present along the gastrointestinal tract and the myenteric plexus. This finding further elucidates the mechanisms for nausea control [52].

Ginger has also been investigated for the treatment of emesis during pregnancy; some clinical trials show that ginger can be valuable as a mean to avoiding vomiting in pregnant women. In a study, pregnant women related relief of nausea and vomiting if they had consumed ginger, while women that had not did not relate so [53]. In another study, ginger could not reduce vomiting, but reduced morning nausea during pregnancy [54].

Another research demonstrated that ginger can actually reduce vomiting and nausea during pregnancy within 3 days of treatment, with effects comparable to those of dimenhydrinate, but with the advantage of exhibiting fewer side effects, such as drowsiness [55]. Before cesarean sections are performed, administration of ginger prior to the surgery reduces the episodes of nausea, but it does not reduce vomiting or the intensity of nausea during the surgery and during the period after it [56].

In these kinds of studies, the only adverse reaction usually linked to ginger consumption is heartburn, and there are no concerns about fetus development. It must be noted, however, that these studies show some disagreement concerning the effectiveness of ginger in preventing nausea during pregnancy, as some studies demonstrated positive effects while other demonstrated no effects at all. This situation was addressed in a recent meta-analysis on this subject, where the authors compiled known information and suggested that ginger might be effective in preventing nausea and emesis, but more studies are needed [57].

Since chemotherapy is a strong factor for nausea development, clinical trials were also performed to evaluate ginger capacity in reducing nausea in cancer patients [58].

Alongside with high protein consumption, ginger reduces emesis induced by chemotherapy. However, ginger's role may not be so critical in this kind of situation, considering the concomitant use of proteins [59].

Another clinical trial demonstrated that ginger preparations administered to cancer patients undergoing chemotherapy make the placebo patients take more antiemetic drugs compared to the patients that receive ginger treatments [60].

Antidiarrhea Property

Studies performed with animals proved the efficacy of ginger in inhibiting intestinal motility, and so it is useful against diarrhea. The whole extract of ginger is capable of reducing acetylcholine induced and electric stimulation induced intestinal contractions in rats; it is suggested that it can act at prejunctional and postjunctional sites to modify enteric motility [61]. An isolated compound, 6-shogaol, was capable of inhibiting carbachol induced accelerated intestinal peristalsis in rats as well, both *in vitro* and *in vivo*. Since contractions could be reverted by atropine, 6-shogaol was thus capable of blocking the cholinergic nervous system and directly inhibited muscle movement [62].

A study demonstrated that an isolated ginger compound, zingerone, was able to block intestinal motility. Both *in vitro* and *in vivo*, colonic motility of rats was reduced when treatment with zingerone preparations was administered. Further investigations showed this happens due to direct effect in the smooth muscle, and it is not related to nervous effects [63]. Another work from the same authors stablished that the same effects of inhibition of colonic motility caused by zingerone also applies to zingerol, but it also involves colonic neurons and not only direct action on the smooth muscle [64].

Anti-Ulcer Property

Gastric protection is another of ginger's application. The anti-ulcer effect has been known for a long time. First studies upon this topic date to 20 years ago. In these past experiments, injections of ulcer-inducing chemicals such as ethanol, chloridric acid, acidic acid, aspirin and indomethacin were less effective in promoting gastric and intestinal ulcers in rats when they were previously treated with ginger extracts. Ginger was also able to prevent gastric lesion in rats due to pylorus ligation. Even without knowing the exact mechanism for the anti-ulcer effect, isolated compounds were tested such as zingiberene, 6-shogaol and 6-gingerol [65-68].

More recently, ginger's efficacy in preventing ulcers and damage caused by colitis can be comparable to major anti-ulcer drugs, such as ranitidine and prednisolone, and is even better than others, like sucralfate [68,69]. Treatment with ginger extract reduces the serum levels of γ-GTP, a marker of cell damage, and promotes mucus production. Ginger's extract also normalizes colonic enzymatic and non-enzymatic oxidative damage defense systems, such as reduced glutathione, catalase and superoxide dismutase, which are also linked to ginger's antioxidant abilities; inflammatory factors, such as PGE2, TNF-α and nitric oxide, also do not have their levels increased. Ginger's efficacy seems to be based upon its antioxidant activity, which prevents free radicals to induce inflammatory response activation. Ginger also promotes thickening of gastric lining [70-73].

Another mechanism is the inhibition of the H+/K+ ATPase present in the parietal cells. Ginger components can actually inhibit this enzyme activity with more efficacy than the proton pump inhibitor lanzoprazole [72].

Ginger extracts reduce ulcers caused by *H. pylori*. This implies that ginger possibly acts as an anti-microbial (as further elaborated in this review). Ginger's extract alone is capable of inhibiting bacterium growth; the effect against *H. pylori* is strengthened when combined with clarithromycin, affecting somewhat resistant bacteria strains [74]. This anti-microbial property exists because ginger's constituents supposedly can acidify the plasma membrane, acidify the intracellular region by blocking H+/K+ ATPase or interfere with some enzyme that regulates membrane permeability [72].

As the effect of gastric protection by ginger extracts is further studied, some authors are already looking into proper applications. A study demonstrated that calcium alginate beads containing ginger extract are efficient not only in preventing gastric damage, but also in curing already existing lesions. The curative effects are possible because the beads ensure ginger stays longer in the stomach without being absorbed and also solve the problem of poor solubility of the ginger extracts in the stomach fluids. This is a very efficient way to administer ginger considering ulcer treatment, and the effects are superior to those of cimetide, as reported by the authors [75].

Anti-Cancer Properties

Cancer is a very spread disease nowadays, which still poses a challenge to public health; ginger can be a useful tool to confront this illness. Several components found in ginger, like gingerols, zingerone and zerumbone, are cited in reviews found in literature as being capable of preventing cancer through various mechanisms: free radical scavenging, blocking of enzymatic pathways and induction of apoptosis [8,76].

Ginger has effects upon several cancer types. It suppresses growth of mammary tumor in rats, prevents proliferation of leukemia cells in culture, reduces the viability of gastric cancer cells and ovarian cancer cells *in vitro* and attenuates carcinogenesis in rat skin [77-81].

Several studies demonstrate the efficacy of ginger extracts and isolated compounds in colon cancer suppression [82-84].

Ginger suppresses tumor growth through various steps. It was reported that ginger extracts reduce the activity levels of some enzymes which increase in cancer conditions, such as alkaline phosphatase, aspartate aminotransferase and alanine aminotransferase, and general metabolic improvement supposedly contributes to cancer prevention [78]. Ginger compounds prevent activation of NF-kappaB, COX-2 and vascular endothelium growth factor pathways, which are all linked to promotion of angiogenesis and, consequently, to tumor development [80, 85]. Ornithine decarboxylase is also a known factor that relates with evolving carcinogenesis; ginger extracts reduce the levels of mRNA referent to this enzyme, thus reducing its expression [77, 79]. Free radicals are also involved in carcinogenesis, as they damage DNA and RNA strands and induce mutations. Ginger reduces lipid peroxidation and enhances the levels of superoxide dismutase, and because of these factors alone, it can reduce tumor development, which shows that the antioxidant properties of ginger are also a crucial factor in carcinogenesis [86].

Tumor necrosis factor-related apoptosis-inducing ligand is promissory in cancer therapy, as it stimulates tumor cells to enter apoptosis; ginger constituents enhance tumor necrosis factor-related apoptosis-inducing ligand activity. This effect is either due to down-regulation of NF-kappaB or to up-regulation of death-receptors 4 and 5; these factors are immersed in long pathways that culminate in apoptosis [79, 84]. Factor NF-kappaB and Bcl proteins are overexpressed in cancerous cells as they prevent apoptosis; ginger treatment can decrease the levels of these factors and also increase the expression of Bax and other factors that promote cell apoptosis [87].

Finally, ginger extracts induce apoptosis and prevent cell growth by other pathways as well. A study showed that ginger prevents DNA synthesis of cancerous cells, as well as interfered with the deregulated mitotic cycle such cells, probably due to inhibition of cyclin-dependant kinases [83].

As there is much research performed with ginger extracts, there are also studies with isolated compounds.

The chemical 6-gingerol was demonstrated to reduce tumor development [88]; it can also antagonize the vascular endothelium growth factor, preventing angiogenesis [85]. This gingerol can also increase TRAIL-induced apoptosis in non-cytotoxic concentrations and increase the expression of death receptors 4 and 5 (as mentioned above) which culminate in activation of p53-induced apoptosis [89]. This compound is responsible for many of ginger's other uses, but as for anti-cancer properties, studies show that it may not be the major chemical. Other constituents, such as galanals A and B were reported as more efficient than 6-gingerol in reducing cancerous cells growth, these can even disrupt mitochondrial function and modify the expression of Bcl-2 and Bax proteins, modifying apoptosis regulation [90], similar effects have also been reported as part of how several terpenoids present in distilled ginger extracts (which contain few gingerols) can prevent cancer and also promote p53-induced apoptosis [91]. Compound 6-paradol and shogaols (such as 6-shogaol, 8-shogaol and 10-shogaol) are also capable of inhibiting cell growth, and shogaols exhibited better capacity than 6-gingerol in achieving this effect [88]. Zerumbone is another chemical already studied. By several pathways, zerumbone also prevents cell growth and induce apoptosis; it also prevents osteoclastogenesis in rats [92, 93].

Cardiovascular System Effects

The cardiovascular system also benefits from ginger chemicals. Ginger's antioxidant properties allow its extract to reduce glucose and cholesterols levels in the blood stream, and its effect over COX allows for blocking of platelet aggregation and preventing of hypotension [5]. A study realized in the United States of America showed that among patients with any cardiovascular disease, 12% used ginger supplements to improve overall health condition [94]. Ginger enhances the cardiovascular system through multiple ways. Studies suggested that the most polar chemicals found in ginger are capable of promoting hypotension due to cholinergic agonism, both in vascular tissue and directly in the heart, while the non-polar constituents induce hypotension due to blocking of Ca^{+2} channels. Nitric oxide release in muscular epithelium can be increased [95,96]. Ginger extracts not only cause hypotension, but can prevent hypertension due to more long-term effects as well.

A study reported that ginger extracts attenuate atherosclerosis; as it is known that ginger possesses a huge amount of antioxidant phenolic compounds, the preventive effect over LDL oxidation is very probable.

Ginger's compounds partially inhibit cholesterol synthesis and interfere with LDL lipoprotein, preventing the aggregation of LDL by macrophages [97].

Recently, some studies demonstrated that ginger extracts inhibit the activity of angiotensin converting enzyme, which helps in elucidating the mechanisms of action responsible for improvement of cardiovascular function [98,99]. A further study reported that compound 6-gingerol is one of the chemicals responsible for inhibition of this enzyme [100].

Platelet aggregation can be prevented with the administration of ginger extracts. Among ginger's several chemical compounds, 6-gingerol and 6-shogaol have been reported as capable of preventing platelet aggregation [101]. Epinephrine and ADP-induced aggregation can be reduced by a single dose of ginger. Ginger extracts also have synergistic effects with nifedipine, boosting its anti-aggregation effect by almost 50%. This happens due to the antioxidant properties of ginger and probably, as ginger inhibits the enzyme COX-2 and prevents inflammations, also due to COX inhibition found in platelets [102, 103].

It is safe enough to use ginger to prevent cardiovascular diseases. Most studies showed the benefits of no more than 10 mg/kg. Bradycardia and hypotension only become dangerous in doses near 50 mg/kg, and heart tissue necrosis only appears in doses of 2500 mg/kg [104].

Biochemical Effects

Biochemical disturbances and the effects that ginger has on them were studied. Several experiments measured the influence ginger has on biochemical standards, such as glucose and lipids levels, body weight and enzymatic activity.

Although there are some discordances among authors, most of them report the beneficial effects of ginger extracts upon blood glucose levels, as they can lower glucose levels (and other related markers) in a diabetes condition [105-112].

It is likely that ginger can reduce hyperglycemia through reduction of oxidative stress [106, 107, 110], improvement of insulin sensitivity due to PPAR-gamma agonism [108], blocking of serotonin receptors [105, 113] or modification of insulin levels and insulin sensitivity [111, 114].

A more specific study revealed that ginger compounds directly affect the myotubes of cells, which improves glucose uptake [109].

Experiments performed in diabetic rats showed that altered hepatic glycolytic enzymes, such as glucokinase and phosphofructokinase, can be partially restored to normality by ginger, possibly due to insulinomimmetic action, which allows glucose to be normally metabolized [112].

As previously mentioned, ginger compounds function as antioxidants; as shown in a study with diabetic rats, every enzyme related to oxidative distress, such as superoxide dismutase, catalase, glutathione peroxidase and glutathione reductase can have its levels normalized by ginger [110].

This affects other enzymes indirectly, such as liver enzymes like aspartate aminotransferase, alanine aminotransferase and gamma glutamyltransferase; these enzymes reflect cell damage, and this damage can be prevented by ginger chemicals, as demonstrated in a study where hepatocytes were subjected to CCL4-induced lipid peroxidation oxidative stress [115].

Glycogen is another factor that is bound to ginger biochemical treatment; in diabetic conditions, the kidney stores glycogen and eventually hypertrophies, as the entrance of glucose in kidneys is not dependent to insulin levels. Ginger modulates carbohydrate blood levels, thus decreasing renal hypertrophy generated by a diabetic condition [107, 112]. Effects on other sites of glycogen deposit, such as liver and muscle, are very controversial.

Ginger's effects on lipids have been investigated. Studies performed in obese rats (either due to high-fat diet, or due to diabetes induction, or due to deficiency in apoliprotein E) with alterations in LDL, cholesterol, phospholipids and triglycerides levels, demonstrated that ginger extracts were able to attenuate the deregulation of overall lipid status [102]. Ginger usage improves cholesterol excretion and prevents the suppressive effect of high fat levels over LDL-receptors [97, 108, 113].

Antioxidant effects of polyphenols found in ginger extract were reported to reduce LDL oxidation and thus prevent atherosclerosis in obese rats [105]. In obese humans, ginger extracts in powder formulations are capable of increasing insulin sensitivity and decreasing levels of LDL and triglycerides [114]. HDL levels do not seem to be affected by ginger compounds, and suffer neither increase nor decrease.

Body weight is also affected by ginger usage. Several researchers concluded that ginger reduces body weight significantly in diabetic rats [105-107, 110, 112].

Studies also showed that ginger extracts were efficient in preventing body weight gain in rats fed with high amounts of fats, possibly due to some interference with adrenergic beta-receptors [108, 113].

Finally, ginger also affects protein levels. In diabetic rats, there is a reduction of blood protein levels, as well as an increase of proteins found in urine. Ginger treatment was able to normalize protein status as shown in some studies [105-108].

Neural Effects

A topic that has been gaining attention in the last years is the neurological protection provided by ginger. Recent research demonstrated that ginger is capable of preventing neural damage from neurotoxic agents and of modifying brain functions. As explained previously, ginger extracts function as a powerful antioxidant agent; this capability is crucial in preventing brain damage. The process of aging accelerates the neurodegenerative evolution of the brain, and part of it happens due to the generation of oxygen free radicals, which damage nervous tissue. Studies found in the scientific literature demonstrated that ginger extracts are capable of protecting nervous cells from oxidative damage; ginger compounds inhibit induced lipid peroxidation by scavenging free radicals or chelating ions that induce such oxidative process, such as Fe^{2+}[116-118]. An unusual study demonstrated that acupuncture applied to rats after induced brain ischemia is capable of improving overall oxidative status in the brain and of restoring cognitive functions. With the aid of ginger extracts, the pharmacopuncture process was reported to be even more efficient than acupuncture alone, as oxidative damage would be reduced even more and cognitive improvement could be seen earlier when compared to acupuncture alone, which suggests ginger might be useful in preventing cognitive impairment after ischemia, but further studies are needed [119].

Ginger also prevents brain damage through other pathways that do not involve direct oxidative damage. A study demonstrated that ginger extracts prevent neurotransmitter depletion caused by excessive treatment with monosodium glutamate in mice. Monosodium glutamate activates receptors which activate Ca^{2+} influx, which in turn causes excessive liberation of neurotransmitters; ginger compounds blocked Ca^{2+} channels, thus preventing ion influx and neurotransmitter depletion [120]. Another study showed that ginger prevents the oxidation of acrylamide, which is responsible for generating several toxic metabolites [121].

The cholinergic system is supposed to be a main area for ginger's actions. A study performed in mice demonstrated that ginger inhibits cholinesterase activity in the brain. Accumulation of acetylcholine could be of value in the treatment of neurodegenerative diseases directly linked to lowering of acetylcholine, such as Alzheimer's disease [118]. In a clinical trial performed with middle-aged women, the attention and cognitive functions of the subjects were significantly improved due to ginger treatment due to its anti-cholinesterasic property [122].

Ginger might also be a future alternative for drug addiction. A study demonstrated that ginger extracts administered to morphine-addicted rats can completely nullify the effects of tolerance, and can prevent to some extension the effects of withdrawal syndrome. The authors further investigated gene expression and detected that ginger prevents the expression of proteins that maintain the structure of Ca^{2+} channels, which are overexpressed in situations of morphine addiction [123].

Anti-Bacterial Properties

The anti-bacterial properties of ginger are responsible for perhaps the most controversial topic found in literature concerning ginger's uses. Some studies say that ginger extracts function as anti-bacterial against several bacteria species, but there are also studies that state the contrary. Not only has the species *Zingiber officinale* been screened for possible anti-microbial activity, but several other plants from the *Zingiberacea* family have also been studied, some presenting anti-bacterial activity, some not [124, 125].

Some bacterium species that were trialed include *E. coli, S. typhi, S. mutans, S. aureaus, S. enteriditis, C. perfringens, P. aeruginosa, P. vulgaris, K. pneumonia, B. subtilis, M. luteus, H. pylori* and *A. baumannii* [13, 74, 125-132]. It is important to note that the solvent used for preparation of the extracts significantly affects the anti-bacterial activity of ginger. For example, the ethanolic extract affects both *E. coli* and *S. typhi*, but the aqueous extract is ineffective against *E. coli*, and is efficient only against *S. typhi* [126]. The scientific literature contains lots of research performed with different extraction solvents, such as water, ethanol, methanol, chloroform and petroleum ether, however, ethanol is the solvent that better extracts the non-polar ginger constituents which are anti-bacterial, and therefore providing better antibacterial capabilities to the extract [126-129]. Still, there are authors that argue that other extracts, such as methanolic ones, possess better anti-bacterial activity [133].

Studies showed that ginger is capable of interacting with other drugs. Ginger compounds modify the resistance profile of *A. baumannii*, making strains of this bacterium sensible to tetracycline where previously they were not [128]. Ginger acts synergistically with clarithromycin, significantly boosting the effects of this drug upon *H. pylori* [74].

On the other hand, academic research also demonstrated that ginger is not such an efficient anti-bacterial. It is reported that none of ginger extracts exhibit anti-bacterial activity, and only its whole oil is able to prevent bacterial growth [13]. Other studies denoted that should ginger extracts inhibit bacterial growth, it would happen only in very high concentrations [134, 135]. Finally, there are studies that showed that ginger extracts by themselves cannot by any means prevent bacterial growth [132, 136, 137]. These studies oppose previous and recent findings about ginger anti-bacterial activity. The applications of ginger concerning this subject remain in discussion.

Anti-Fungal Properties

Ginger has potential not only as an anti-bacterial, as it is also capable of inhibiting fungal growth. Every study present in the literature that shows evaluation of fungal growth does so by means of the standard disc diffusion technique. Inhibition of growth has been confirmed in strains of *Rhizopus solani, Candida albicans, Malassezia furfur, Alternaria citri, Aspergillus niger, Aspergillus flavus, Fusarium roseum, Aspergillus fumigatus, Fusarium nivale, Rhizopus stolonifer, Penicillium notatum* and several others. There is a minor disagreement among authors about the extension of ginger's anti-fungal activity. While some report absolute inhibition, even superior to known antibiotics, others report only a slight inhibition. This is acceptable, however, since the fungi used in most experiments tend to be different. Nonetheless, it is a fact that every author confirms the anti-fungal effects of ginger [138-147].

Some fungi, such as species of *Fusarium* and *Aspergillus*, can produce mycotoxins which are common contaminants found in food. The growth inhibition of these fungi prevents the contamination of foods [148, 149] and therefore directly reduces the production of mycotoxins [150]. Ginger oil has been experimentally proven as capable of preventing the production of fumonisins B_1 and B_2 *in vitro* by *Fusarium verticillioides*, as well as preventing fungal growth *per se* by inhibiting ergosterol production [151]. The anti-fungal property of ginger is also valuable in improving the shelf-time of foods. Grapes fumigated in ginger oil have 6 more viable days in storage. Ginger also reduces the oxidative status and the microbial content in stored smoked fish [141, 152].

In a study performed with multi-drug resistant *C. albicans*, ginger ethyl acetate extract was effective as anti-fungal, preventing the growth of the fungi where common drugs usually would not [153].

Mostly, the known compounds gingerols and zingiberen are reported to be responsible for the anti-fungal activity shown by ginger. A study suggested this activity can also be due to proteins found in the rhizome [154].

Anti-Parasitary Properties

Another uses for ginger described in scientific literature are the control of some vectors of parasitical diseases and the control of the parasites themselves. Some reports attest ginger extracts are capable of killing the snail *Lymnaea acuminata*, the vector for *Fasciola* species that are endemic in India. Depending on the concentration of the extract being used, the larvae which parasite the snail can be killed leaving the snail unaffected; by leaving the snail alive, less impact upon ecological environments happens [155, 156].

As well as the whole extract, ginger's isolated compounds also exhibit larvicidal activity. All major gingerols, like 6-gingerol, 8-gingerol and 10-gingerol and 6-shogaol are capable of successfully killing *Angiostrongylus cantonensis* larvae bred in culture dishes [157].

Both crude ginger and its extract are efficient against helminthic infections. An *in vivo* study demonstrated that ginger reduces the viability and development of several gastrointestinal nematodes in faeces, such as *Haemonchus contortus*, *Trichostrongylus colubriformis*, *Trichostrongylus axei*, *Oesophagostomum columbianum*, *Strongyloides papillosus* and *Trichurisovis* [158]. *In vivo* studies performed with mice infected with *Schistossoma mansoni* showed that treatment with ginger extracts is capable of reducing worm development and egg count, and it also improves the status of hepatic markers which enter in imbalance due to fibrosis caused by the parasites, such as enzymes aspartate aminotransferase and alanine aminotransferase [159, 160].

Against insects, ginger oleoresin is capable of inhibiting *S. obliqua* larvae growth and it shows antifeedant activity as well, preventing the larvae from feeding upon leaves treated with it. Compounds derived from the oleoresin also inhibit growth and feeding, but to a lesser extent, which suggests the integrity of the oleoresin is necessary for its action, probably due to synergistic effects of all of its chemicals that must be present altogether [138].

Preventing Intoxications

Several studies demonstrated the efficacy of ginger in preventing various kinds of intoxications that cause oxidative damage. Chemicals such as carbon tetrachloride and acrylamide [115, 121], heavy metals such as lead and cadmium [161-163], drugs such as non-steroidal anti-inflammatories [164] and antibiotics [165] and organophosphate pesticides such as fenitrothion [162] induce oxidative stress, reducing the levels of protective enzymes such as superoxide dismutase, catalase and glutathione transferase.

Ginger treatment normalizes the protective enzyme levels and prevents lipid peroxidation that would further increase the oxidative damage caused in different biological systems [121, 161-165].

Ethanol is a very common drug that also disrupts the oxidative balance of the human body when ingested in excess due to its conversion to acetaldehyde (which generates free radicals), damaging kidneys and liver. Ginger treatment prevents the damage by restoring the oxidative status to normal, which can be further proven by the normalizing of liver biomarkers, such as alanine aminotransferase, aspartate aminotransferase, gamma glutamyltranspeptidase and alkaline phosphatase, which is possible even under cirrhosis conditions [110, 166-169].

TOXICITY

Natural products, if misused, can cause allergic and toxic reactions. Contaminants can also be present in formulations supposedly harmless, such as heavy metals, pesticides or other drugs. As any other plant product, ginger must be used with caution. Besides, pharmacological/toxicological interactions with other drugs can easily occur [2]. Therefore, there are some studies that demonstrated toxicity caused by ginger to some extent.

Considering biochemical parameters, a study showed that doses up to 100 mg/kg of ginger in normal rats are inefficient in causing any changes in blood glucose [170]. In higher doses, up to 500 mg/kg, levels of some enzymes are affected. Heart lactate dehydrogenase, aspartate aminotransferase and alanine aminotransferase levels only slightly increase. Alkaline phosphatase activity as well as serum proteins levels remain unchanged. Even on higher doses, ginger does not affect the liver [171].

Blood standards are modified due to high doses of ginger. Reduction of hemoglobin concentrations is verified in healthy rats exposed to 500 mg/kg of ginger. The reduction is not enough to change any body function, though. Hematocrit remains unchanged at this dose [171].

As for cardiovascular parameters, 100 mg/kg of ginger dried extract does not affect platelet aggregation, heart rate, nor blood pressure [170]. However, higher doses can be dangerous; 500 mg/kg of ginger are enough to produce reduction in both systolic and diastolic pressures, as well as induce drops in heart rate and blood pressure. Swelling of heart tissue also occurs [104].

There is not enough data available that allow solid conclusions about the teratogenic effects of ginger. In humans, studies reported that no abortions occur and infants do not show malformations when pregnant women were treated with ginger [54].

In pregnant rats, a study stated that ginger does not demonstrate any toxic effects, neither for mother nor fetus. In the concentration of 1000 mg/kg, some minor skeletal malformations appear, but they are not statistically relevant [172]. Contradictory to this study, use of ginger extracts by pregnant rats in the same concentration induced significant abortion and fetus resorption as reported by other authors [173, 174].

These antagonisms demonstrate that more studies are needed to establish the possibility of teratogenic effects related to ginger consumption.

Upon human semen, ginger extract in concentrations up to 0.6% reduces spermatozoid count and motility in a dose-dependent manner, until total immobility of spermatozoids [175].

Some studies performed with mutant strains of *S. typhimurium* stated that ginger constituents have mutagenic activities. The compounds 6-gingerol and 6-shogaol were reported as mutagenic, while zingiberene was not [176, 177]. This information could be troublesome, but considering that these studies are old, the fact that ginger has been for long used safely, and that the great number of recent studies performed with these compounds demonstrate their preventive effect against mutagenicity, cancer development due to ginger use is not a concern. This information should at least stand for the lack of toxicity effects involving mutagenicity.

Despite the fact that several studies demonstrated that ginger extracts have at least some minor toxic effects, it is quite safe to use them in experiments. Various researches performed upon rats demonstrated that the LD_{50} is reached at very high doses. Mice are killed when exposed to ginger doses higher than 1000 mg/kg. In other studies, ginger is far more harmless, where LD_{50} is achieved at doses of 10000 mg/kg [31, 112, 178, 179].

However, a sub-chronic study carried for 35 days with normal rats under ginger treatment in high doses opposed other findings about ginger toxicity.

Doses of 2000 mg/kg of ginger, except for a slight decrease of both lactate dehydrogenase and body weight, could not cause any changes in biochemical or hematological parameters. Such contradiction proves the necessity for more studies concerning the safety of ginger for further elucidation of its toxic effects [180].

It must be noted that many plant preparations used popularly are not subjected to a rigorous quality control and might also contain contaminants that are possibly toxic. A study showed that the heavy metals lead, cadmium, mercury and arsenic can be detected in ginger rhizomes growing in Asia [181]. In this manner, toxicity might not be caused by ginger *per se*.

CONCLUSION

The contribution of this review to future studies is to expand the basis of research compilations about effects of ginger's rhizome essential oil and its extracts found in literature, including both the previously and well-documented researches and the newer ones that are receiving increased attention. There are plenty of studies about isolated chemical compounds, but recent researches show that not just a single chemical found in ginger, such as 6-gingerol and zingiberene, but several acting in synergism are responsible for the effects described in this review, even though 6-gingerol is often reported as a main compound responsible alone for many of ginger's properties.

Several beneficial and applicable effects of ginger have already been vastly studied and documented, such as the antioxidant, anti-nausea and anti-inflammatory properties. Recent researches demonstrate that ginger possesses still other applications, and it could be useful in the treatment of cardiovascular diseases, intoxications and other metabolic problems.

It is important to state that the antioxidant activity of ginger's phenolics is the main property responsible for the majority of the other effects described in this review.

Ginger is an extensively studied plant that has been used for ages for the treatment of the most varied illnesses, being relatively safe for use. Still, some studies demonstrated that high dosages lead to some physiological alterations. More studies are still needed in order to further elucidate ginger's safety, but it is overall safe for use.

REFERENCES

[1] Kemper, K.J. (1999). *Longwood Herbal Task Force.* 3: 1-18.

[2] Veiga Junior, V.F., A.C. Pinto and M.A.M. Maciel (2005) *Quim. Nova.*28 (3): 519-528.

[3] Ali, B.H., G. Blunden, M.O. Tanira,and A. Nemmar (2007) *Food Chem. Toxicol.* 46: 409–420.

[4] Chrubasik, S., M.H. Pittlercand B.D. Roufogalis (2004) *Phytomedicine.* 12: 684–701.

[5] Nicoll, R. and M.Y. Henein (2007) *Letters to the Editor.* 408-409.

[6] Bryer, E. (2005) *J. Midwifery Wom. Heal.* 50 (1): e1-e3.

[7] Ernst, E. and M.H. Pittler (2000) *Brit. J. Anaesth.* 84 (3): 367-371.

[8] Shukla, Y. and M. Singh (2006) *Food Chem. Toxicol.* 45: 683–690.

[9] Zancan, K.C., M.O.M. Marques, A.J. Petenate,and M.A.A. Meireles (2002) *J. Supercrit. Fluid.* 24: 57–76.

[10] Justo, O.R., Â.M. Moraes, G.P.M. Barreto, A.Z. Mercadante,and P.T.V. Rosa (2008) *Quim. Nova.*31 (7): 1699-1705.

[11] Jaafar, H.Z.E., A. Ghasemzadehand A. Rahmat (2010) *Molecules.* 15: 4324-4333.

[12] Nishimura, O. (1995) *J. Agric. Food Chem.*43: 2941-2945.

[13] Singh, G., I.P.S. Kapoor, P. Singh, C.S. de Heluani, M.P. de Lampasona,and C.A.N. Catalan (2008) *Food Chem. Toxicol.* 46: 3295–3302.

[14] Pereira, R.C.B., A.J.R. Silva, A.L.S. Barbosa,and A.U.O. Sabaa-Srur (2007) *Rev. Univ. Rural, Sér. Ci. da Vida.* 27 (1): 10-20.

[15] Dabague, I.C.M., C. Deschamps, A.F. Mógor, A.P. Scheer,and L. Côcco (2011) *Rev. Bras. Pl. Med.* 13 (1): 79-84.

[16] Asghari, G. and P. Anasori (2008) *Research in Pharmaceutical Sciences.* 3(1): 59-63.

[17] Jaafar, H.Z.E. and A. Ghasemzadeh (2011) *Int. J. Mol. Sci.*12:1101-1114.

[18] Maia, N.B., O.A.Bovi and F.R. Duarte (1991) *Bragantina, Campinas.* 50 (1): 83-92.

[19] Stoilova, I., A. Krastanov, A. Stoyanova, P. Denev,and S. Gargova (2006) *Food Chem.* 102: 764–770.

[20] Ajith, T.A., V. Nivithaand S. Usha (2007) *Food Chem. Toxicol.* 45: 921–927.

[21] Ajith, T.A., U. Hemaand M. S. Aswathy (2007) *Food Chem. Toxicol.* 45: 2267–2272.

[22] Ko, J.K. and Leung, C.C. (2010) *J. Gastroen. Hepatol.* 25: 1861-1869.
[23] Ramadan, G., M.A. Al-Kahtaniand W.M. El-Sayed (2011) *Inflammation* 34 (4): 291-301.
[24] Damu, A.G., P.C. Kuo, C.Y. Cherng, J.F. Jeng, C.M. Teng, E.J. Lee,and T.S. Wu (2004) *Arch. Pharm. Res.* 28 (5): 518-528.
[25] Ippoushi, K., K. Azuma, H. Ito, H. Horie,and H. Higashio (2003) *Life Sci.* 73: 3427–3437.
[26] Chung, D.M., S.M.N. Uddin and J.K. Kim (2013) *Korean J. Environ. Biol.* 31 (4) 376-382.
[27] Grzanna, R., L. Lindmarkand C.G. Frondoza (2005) *J. Med. Food.* 8 (2): 125–132.
[28] Breemen, R.B., Y. Tao and W. Li (2011) *Fitoterapia* 82: 38-43.
[29] Raji, Y., U. S. Udoh, O.O. Oluwadara, O.S. Akinsomisoye, O.Awobajo,and K.Adeshoga (2002) *Afr. J. Biomed. Res.* 5: 121–124.
[30] Thomson, M., K.K. Al-Qattan, S.M. Al-Sawan, M.A. Alnaqeeb, I. Khan,and M. Ali (2002) *Prostag.,Leukotr. Ess.* 67 (6): 475-478.
[31] Ojewole, J.A.O. (2006) *Phytother. Res.* 20: 764–772.
[32] Shimoda, H., S.J. Shan, J. Tanaka, A. Seki, J.W. Seo, N. Kasajima, S. Tamura, Y. Ke,and N. Murakami (2010) *J. Med. Food.* 13 (1): 156–162.
[33] Penna, S.C., M.V. Medeiros, F.S.C. Aimbire, H.C.C. Faria-Neto, J.A.A. Sertié,and R.A.B. Lopes-Martins (2003) *Phytomedicine.* 10: 381–385.
[34] Atashak, S., M. Peeri, M.A. Azarbayjani, S.R. Stannard,and M.M. Haghighi (2011) *J. Sport Sci. Med.* 10: 685-691.
[35] Lantz, R.C., G.J. Chen, M. Sarihan, A.M. Sólyom, S.D. Jolad,and B.N. Timmermann (2007) *Phytomedicine.* 14: 123–128.
[36] Jung, H.W., C.-H. Yoon, K.M. Park, H.S. Han,and Y.-K. Park (2009) *Food Chem. Toxicol.* 47: 1190–1197.
[37] Li, X.H., K.C.Y. McGrath, S. Nammi, A.K. Heather,and B.D. Roufogalis (2012) *Basic Clin. Pharmacol.* 110: 238-244.
[38] Zhou, H.-L., Y.-M. Deng and Q.-M. Xie (2005) *J. Ethnopharmacol.* 105: 301–305.
[39] Young, H.-Y., Y.-L. Luo, H.-Y. Cheng, W.-C. Hsieh, J.-C. Liao,and W.-H. Peng (2004) *J. Ethnopharmacol.* 96: 207–210.
[40] Tripathi, S., K.G. Maier, D. Bruch,and D.S. Kittur (2006) *J. Surg. Res.* 138: 209–213.
[41] Ahui, M.L.B., P. Champy, A. Ramadan, L.P. Van, L. Araujo, K.B. André, S. Diem, D. Damotte, S. Kati-Coulibaly, M.A. Offoumou, M. Dy, N. Thieblemont,and A. Herbelin (2008) *Int. Immunopharmacol.* 8: 1626–1632.

[42] Chen, B.-H., P.-Y. Wu, K.-M. Chen, T.-F. Fu, H.-M. Wang,and C.-Y. Chen (2009) *J. Nat. Prod.* 72 (5):950–953.

[43] Lee, H.Y., S.H. Park, M. Lee, H.J. Kim, S.H. Ryu, N.D. Kim, B.Y. Hwang, J.T. Hong, S.B. Han,and Y. Kim (2012) *Brit. J. Pharmacol.* 167: 128-140.

[44] Haghighi, M., A. Khalvat, T. Toliat,and S. Jallaei (2005) *Arch. Iran. Med.* 8: 267-271.

[45] Wigler, I., I. Grotto, D. Caspi,and M. Yaron (2003) *Osteoarthr. Cartilage.*11: 783–789.

[46] Ozgoli, G., M. Goliand F. Moattar (2008) *J. Altern. Complem. Med.* 15 (2): 129-132.

[47] Black, C.D., M.P. Herring, D.J. Hurley,and P.J. O'Connory (2009) *J. Pain.* 11 (9): 894-903.

[48] Mowrey, D.B. and D.E. Clayson (1982) *Lancet.* 655-657.

[49] Lien, H.-C., W.M. Sun, Y.-H. Chen, H. Kim, W. Hasler,and C. Owyang (2002) *Am. J. Physiol-Gastr. L.* 284: G481–G489.

[50] Sharma, S.S., V. Kochupillai, S.K. Gupta, S.D. Seth,and Y.K. Gupta (1997) *J. Ethnopharmacol.* 57: 93–96.

[51] Haksar, A., A. Sharma, R. Chawla, R. Kumar, R. Arora, S. Singh, J. Prasad, M. Gupta, R.P. Tripathi, M.P. Arora, F. Islam,and R.K. Sharma (2006) *Pharmacol. Biochem. Be.* 84: 179–188.

[52] Pertz, H.H., J. Lehmann, R.R. Ehrang,and S. Elz (2011) *Planta Med.* 77: 973-978.

[53] Fischer-Rasmussen, W., S.K. Kjser, C. Dahl,and U. Asping (1990) *Eur. J. Obstet. Gyn. R. B.* 38: 19-24.

[54] Willetts, K.E., A. Ekangakiand John, A.E.D.E.N. (2003) *Aust. NZ. J. Obstet. Gyn.* 43: 139–144.

[55] Pongrojpaw, D., C. Somprasitand A. Chanthasenanont (2007) *J. Med. Assoc. Thai.*90 (9): 1703-1709.

[56] Kalava, A., S.J. Darji, A. Kalstein, J.M. Yarmush, J.S. Cola,and J. Weinberg (2013) *Eur. J. Obstet. Gyn. R. B.* 169: 184-188.

[57] Thomsom, M., R. Corbin and L. Leung (2014) *J. Am. Board Fam. Med.* 27 (1): 115-122.

[58] Hickok, J.T., J.A. Roscoe, G.R. Morrow,and J.L. Ryan (2007) *Supportive Cancer Therapy.* 4 (4): 247-250.

[59] Levine, M.E., M.G. Gillis, S.Y. Koch, A.C. Voss, R.M. Stern,and K.L. Koch (2008) *J. Altern. Complem. Med.* 14 (5): 545–551.

[60] Ryan, J.L., C.E. Heckler, J.A. Roscoe, S.R. Dakhil, J. Kirshner, P.J. Flynn, J.T. Hickok,and G.R. Morrow (2012) *Support. Care Cancer* 20 (7): 1479-1489.

[61] Borrelli, F., R. Capassoa, A. Pinto,and A.A. Izzo (2003) *Life Sci.* 74: 2889–2896.

[62] Hashimoto, K., K. Satoh, P. Murata, B. Makino, I. Sakakibara, Y. Kase, A. Ishige, M. Higuchi,and H. Sasaki (2002) *Planta Med.* 68: 936-939.

[63] Iwami, M., T. Shiina, H. Hirayama, T. Shima, T. Takewaki,and Y. Shimizu (2010) *J. Nat. Med.* 65: 89–94.

[64] Iwami, M., T.Shiina, H. Hirayama,and Y. Shimizu (2011) *Biomed. Res.* 32 (2): 181-185.

[65] Yamahara, J., M. Mochizuki, H. Q. Rong, H. Matsuda,and H. Fujimura (1988) *J. Ethnopharmacol.* 23:299-304.

[66] Al-Yahya, M.A., S. Rafatullah, J. S. Mossa, A.M. Ageel, N.S. Parmar,and M. Tariq (1988) *Am. J. Chinese Med.* 17 (1-2): 5 1–56.

[67] Yoshikawa, M., M. Yamaguchi, K. Kunimi, H. Matsuda, Y. Okuno, J. Yamahara,and N. Murakami (1994) *Chem. Pharm. Bull.* 42 (6):1226-1230.

[68] Minaiyan, M., A. Ghannadiand A. Karimzadeh (2006) *DARU.* 14 (2): 97-101.

[69] Rashidian, A., S. Mehrzadi, A.R. Ghannadi, P. Mahzooni, S. Sadr,and M. Minaiyan (2014) *J. Integr. Med.* 12 (2): 115-120.

[70] El-Abhara, H.S., L.N.A. Hammadand H.S. Abdel Gawad (2008) *J. Ethnopharmacol.* 118: 367–372.

[71] Khushtar, M., V. Kumar, K. Jared,and U. Bhandari (2009) *Indian J. Pharm. Sci.* 71(5): 554-558.

[72] Nanjundaiah, S.M., H.N.M. Annaiahand S.M. Dharmesh (2009) *Evid.-Based. Compl. Alt.* 2011: 1-13.

[73] Wang, Z., J. Hasegawa, X. Wang, A. Matsuda, T. Tokuda, N. Miura,and T. Watanabe (2011) *Yonago Acta Med.* 54: 11-19.

[74] Nostro, A., L. Cellini, S. Di Bartolomeo, M.A. Cannatelli, E. Di Campli, F. Procopio, R. Grande, L. Marzio,and V. Alonzo (2006) *Phytother. Res.* 20: 187–190.

[75] Singh, P.K. and I.P. Kaur (2011) *J. Drug Target.* 19 (9): 741-751.

[76] Surh, Y.-J. (2002) *Food Chem. Toxicol.* 40: 1091–1097.

[77] Katiyar, S.K., R. Agarwal and H. Mukhtar (1996) *Cancer Res.* 56: 1023-1030.

[78] Nagasawa, H., K. Watanabe and H. Inatomi (2002) *Am. J. Chinese Med.* 30 (2-3): 195–205.

[79] Ishiguro, K., T. Ando, O. Maeda, N. Ohmiya, Y. Niwa, K. Kadomatsu, H. Goto (2007) *Biochem. Bioph. Res. Co.* 362: 218–223.

[80] Rhode, J., S. Fogoros, S. Zick, H. Wahl, K.A. Griffith, J. Huang,and J.R. Liu (2007) *BMC Complem. Alter. M.*7 (44): 1-9.

[81] Omoregie, S.N., F.O. Omoruyi, V.F. Wright, L. Jones,and P.V. Zimba (2013) *J. Med. Food* 16 (7) 647-655.

[82] Manju, V. and N. Nalini (2005) *Clin. Chim. Acta.* 358: 60–67.

[83] Abdullah, S., S.A.Z. Abidin, N.A. Murad, S. Makpol, W.Z.W. Ngah,and Y.A.M. Yusof (2010) *Afr. J. Biochem. Res.* 4(4): 134-142.

[84] Yodkeeree, S., B. Sung, P. Limtrakul,and B.B. Aggarwal (2009) *Cancer Res.* 69 (16): 6581-6589.

[85] Kim, J.-K. E.-C., Min T.-Y. Kim, S.-J. Lee, H.-O. Yang, S. Han, Y.-M. Kim,and Y.-G. Kwon (2005) *Biochem. Bioph. Res. Co.* 335: 300–308.

[86] Yusof, Y.A.M., N. Ahmad, S. Das, S. Sulaiman,and N.A. Murad (2008) *Afr. J. Trad.*6 (1): 87–93.

[87] Elkady, A.I., O.A. Abuzinadah, N.A. Baeshen,and T.R. Rahmy (2012) *J. Biomed. Biotechnol.* doi:10.1155/2012/614356.

[88] Sang, S., J. Hong, H. Wu, J. Liu, C.S. Yang, M.-H. Pan, V. Badmaev,and C.-T. Ho (2009) *J. Agr. Food Chem.* 57(22): 10645–10650.

[89] Lee, D.H., D.W. Kim, C.H. Jung, Y.J. Lee,and D. Park (2014) *Toxicol. Appl. Pharmacol.* doi:10.1016/j.taap.2014.06.030.

[90] Miyoshi, N., Y. Nakamura, Y. Ueda, M. Abe, Y. Ozawa, K. Uchida,and T. Osawa (2003) *Cancer Lett.* 199: 113–119.

[91] Liu, Y., R.J. Whelan, B.R. Pattnaik, K. Ludwig, E. Subudhi, H. Rowland, N. Claussen, N. Zucker, S. Uppal, D.M. Kushner, M. Felder, M.S. Patankar,and A. Kapur (2012) *Plos One* 7 (12).

[92] Sung, B., A. Murakami, B.O. Oyajobi,and B.B. Aggarwal (2009) *Cancer Res.* 69 (4): 1477-1484.

[93] Murakami, A., D. Takahashi, T. Kinoshita, K. Koshimizu, H.W. Kim, A. Yoshihiro, Y. Nakamura, S. Jiwajinda, J. Terao,and H. Ohigashi (2002) *Carcinogenisis.* 23 (5):795-802.

[94] Yeh, G.Y., R.B. Davis and R.S. Phillips (2006) *Am. J. Cardiol.* 98: 673–680.

[95] Ghayur, M.N., M. Phil and A.H. Gilani (2004) *J. Cardiovasc. Pharm.* 45 (1):74–80.

[96] Ghayur, M.N., A.H. Gilani, M.B. Afridi,and P. J. Houghton (2005) *Vasc. Pharmacol.* 43: 234–241.

[97] Fuhrman, B., M. Rosenblat, T. Hayek, R. Coleman,and M. Aviram (2000) *J. Nutr. 1*124-1131.
[98] Akinyemi, A.J., A.O. Ademiluyiand G. Oboh (2013) *J. Med. Food* 16 (7): 641-646.
[99] Akinyemi, A.J., A.O. Ademiluyiand G. Oboh (2014) *J. Med. Food* 17 (3): 317-323.
[100] Liu, Q., J. Liu, H. Guo, S. Sun, S. Wang, Y. Zhang, S. Li,and Y. Qiao (2013) *Planta Med.* 79: 332-326.
[101] Liao, Y.R., Y.L. Leu, Y.Y. Chan, P.C. Kuo,and T.S. Yu (2012) *Molecules* 17: 8928-8937.
[102] Bordia, A., S.K. Vermaand K.C. Srivastava (1997) *Prostag. Leukotr. Ess.* 56 (5): 379-384.
[103] Young, H.-Y., J.-C. Liao, Y.-S. Chang, Y.-L. Luo, M.-C. Lu,and W.-H. Peng (2006) *Am. J. Chinese Med.* 34 (4): 545–551.
[104] Elkhishin, I.A.and I.A. Awwad (2009) *Mansoura J. Forensic Med. Clin. Toxicol.*17 (2): 109-127.
[105] Al-Amin, Z.M., M. Thomson, K.K. Al-Qattan, R. Peltonen-Shalaby,and M. Ali (2006) *Brit. J. Nutr.* 96: 660–666.
[106] Al-Qattan, K., M. Thomson and M. Ali (2008) *e-SPEN, the European e-Journal of Clinical Nutrition and Metabolism*. 3: e62-e71.
[107] Shanmugam, K.R., Ch. Ramakrishana, K. Mallikarjuna,and K.S. Reddy (2009) *Asian J. Exp. Sci.* 23 (1): 127-134.
[108] Nammi, S., S. Sreemantulaand B.D. Roufogalis (2009) *Basic Clin. Pharmacol.* 104*:* 366–373.
[109] Noipha, K., S. Ratanachaiyavongand P. Ninla-aesong (2010*) Diabetes Res. Clin. Pr.* 89: e22-e26.
[110] Shanmugam, K.R., K. Mallikarjuna, K. Nishanth, C.H. Kuo,and K.S. Reddy (2011) *Food Chem.* 124: 1436–1442.
[111] Eyo, J.E., J.C. Ozougwuand P.C. Echi (2011) *Med. J. Islamic World Acad. Sci.* 19(3): 121-126.
[112] Abdulrazaq, N.B., M.M. Cho, N.N. Win, R. Zaman,and M.T. Rahman (2011) *Brit. J. Nutr.* 1-8.
[113] Malik, Z.A. and P.L. Sharmaa (2011) *Int. J. Pharmacol.* 7 (8): 801-812.
[114] Mahluji, S., V.E. Attari, M. Mobasseri, L. Payahoo, A. Ostadrahimi,and S.E.J. Golzari (2013) *Int. J. Food Sci. Nutr.* 64 (6): 682-686.
[115] Atta, A.H., T.A. Elkoly, S.M. Mouneir, G. Kamel, N.A. Alwabel,and S. Zaher (2010) *Indian J. Pharm. Sci.* 72(5): 564-570.
[116] Ajith, T.A. (2010) *Indian J. Clin. Biochem.* 25(1:) 67-73.

[117] Oboh, G., A.J. Akinyemiand A.O. Ademiluyi (2010) *Exp. Toxicol. Pathol.* 64: 31–36.

[118] Oboh, G., A.O. Ademiluyiand A.J. Akinyemi (2010) *Exp. Toxicol. Pathol.* 1-5.

[119] Jittiwat, J. and J. Wattanathorn (2012) *J. Acupunct. Meridian Stud.* 5 (6): 295-300.

[120] Waggas, A.M. (2009) *Pak. J. Biol. Sci.* 12 (3): 201-212.

[121] El-Tantawi, H.G.M. (2007) *Egyp. J. Histol.* 30 (2): 325-336.

[122] Saenghong, N., J.Wattanathorn, S.Muchimapura, T. Tongun, N. Piyavhatkul, C. Banchonglikitkul,and T. Kajsongkram (2011) *Evid.-Based. Compl. Alt.*2012: 1-9.

[123] Mahani, F.D., S.E. Mahani, G. Komeili, V. Sheibani,and L. Zare (2012) *J. Ethnopharmacol.* 141: 901-907.

[124] Habsah, M., M. Amran, M.M. Mackeen, N.H. Lajis, H. Kikuzaki, N. Nakatani, A.A. Rahman, Ghafarand A.M. Ali (2000) *J. Ethnopharmacol.* 72: 403–410.

[125] Sayyad, S.F. and S.R. Chaudhari (2010) *J. Curr. Pharmaceut. Res.* 4 (1): 1-3.

[126] Ekweyne, U.N. and N.N. Elegalam (2005) *Int. J. Mol. Med. Adv. Sci.* 1 (4): 411-416.

[127] Azu, N.C., R.A. Onyeagba, O. Nworie,and J. Kalu (2007) *Internet J. Trop. Med.* 3 (2): 1-8.

[128] Azu, N.C. and R.A. Onyeagba (2007) *Internet J. Trop. Med.* 3 (2): 1-8.

[129] Sunilson, J.A.J., R. Suraj, G. Rejitha, K. Anandarajagopal, A.V.A.G. Kumari,and P. Promwichit (2009) *Am. J. Food Technol.* 1-8.

[130] Wang, H.-M., C.-Y. Chen, H.-A. Chen, W.-C. Huang, W.-R. Lin, T.-C. Chen, C.-Y. Lin, H.-J. Chien, P.-L. Lu, C.-M. Lin,and Y.-H. Chen (2010) *Phytotherapy Res.* 24: 1825–1830.

[131] Auta, K.I., A.A. Galadima, J.U. Bassey, O.D. Olowoniji, O.O. Moses,and A.B. Yako (2011) *Res. J. Biol. Sci.* 6 (1): 37-39.

[132] Rahman, S., A.K. Parvez, R. Islam,and M.H. Khan (2011) *Ann. Clin. Microbiol. Antimicrob.* 10 (10): 1-4.

[133] Gull, I., M. Saeed, H. Shaukat, S.M. Aslam, Z.Q. Samra,and A.M. Athar (2012) *Ann. Clin. Microbiol. Antimicrob.* 11 (8).

[134] Hoffmann, F.L., S.J.F. Souza, C.H. Garcia-Cruz, T.M. Vinturim,and A.L. Dutra (1999) *B.CEPPA*.17 (1): 11-20.

[135] Hammer, K.A., C.F. Carson and T.V. Riley (1999) *J. Appl. Microbiol.* 86: 985–990.

[136] Onyeagba, R.A., O.C. Ugbogu, C.U. Okeke,and O. Iroakasi (2004) *Afr. J. Biotechnol.* 3 (10): 552-554.
[137] Melendez, P.A. and V.A. Capriles (2006) *Phytomedicine.* 13: 272–276.
[138] Agarwal, M., S. Walia, S. Dhingra,and B.P.S. Khambay (2001) *Pest Manag. Sci.* 57: 289-300.
[139] Bruni, R., G. Sacchetti, S. Maietti, M. Muzzoli, M. Scaglianti, S. Manfredini,and M. Radice (2004) *Food Chem.* 91: 621–632.
[140] Hassan, M.M., S.P. Chowdhury, S. Alam, B. Hossain,and M.S. Alam (2005) *Pakistan Journal of Biological Sciences.* 8 (9): 1284-1289.
[141] Tripathi, P., N.K. Dubeyand A.K. Shukla (2007) *World J. Microb. Biot.* 24: 39–46.
[142] Bansod, S. and M. Rai (2008) *World J. Med. Sci.* 3 (2): 81-88.
[143] Banso, A. (2009) *Afr. J. Microbiol. Res.* 3(9): 487-490.
[144] Ayodele, S.M., E.M. Ilonduand N.C. Onwubolu (2009) *Afr. J. Plant Sci.* 3 (6): 139-141.
[145] Sharma, R., G. Sharma and M. Sharma (2011) *J. Med. Plants Res.* 5 (32): 6987-6990.
[146] Singh, H., G. Fairs and M. Syarhabil (2011) *International Conference on Biomedical Engineering and Technology.* 11: 1-6.
[147] Tagoe, D.N.A., H.D. Nyarkoand R. Akpaka (2011) *Res. J. Med. Plants.* 5 (3): 281-287.
[148] Nguefack, J., V. Leth, P.H.A. Zollo,and S.B. Mathur (2004) *Int. J. Food Microbiol.* 94: 329–334.
[149] Kumar, R., N.K. Dubey, O. P. Tiwari, Y.B. Tripathi,and K.K. Sinha (2007) *J. Sci. Food Agr.* 87: 1737–1742.
[150] Ali, S.E., A.A. El–Shaffey, M.E.Selim, K.F. El-Massry,and B.A. Sabry (2010) *J. Biologically Active Prod. Nature.* 1 (1): 81-96.
[151] Ribeiro, M.M.G.Y., R. Grespan, C. Y. Kohiyama, F.D. Ferreira, S.A.G. Mossini, E.L. Silva, B.A. Abreu Filho, J.M.G. Mikcha,and M. Machinski Junior (2013) *Food Chem.* 141: 3147-3152.
[152] Kumolu-Johnson, C.A. and P.E. Ndimele (2011) *Asian J. Biol. Sci.* 4 (7): 532-539.
[153] Khan, R., M. Zakir, S.H. Afaq, A. Latif,and A.U. Khan (2010) *J. Infect. Dev. Ctries.*4 (5): 292-300.
[154] Wang, H. and T. Bun (2005) *Biochem. Biophy. Res. Co.* 336: 100–104.
[155] Sunita, K. and D.K. Singh (2011) *J. Parasitol. Res.* 2011: 1-7.
[156] Singh, V., P. Kumar, V.K. Singh,and D.K. Singh (2010) *Nat. Sci.* 2 (10): 1148-1154.

[157] Lin, R.-J., C.-Y. Chen, L.-Y. Chung,and C.-M. Yen (2010) *Acta Trop.* 115: 69–76.
[158] Iqbal, Z., M. Lateef, M.S. Akhtar, M.N. Ghayur,and A.H. Gilani (2006) *J. Ethnopharmacol.* 106: 285–287.
[159] Mostafa, O.M.S., R.A. Eidand M.A. Adly (2011) *Parasitol. Res.* 109: 395-403.
[160] Aly, H.F. and M.M. Mantawy (2013) *Parasitol. Int.* 62: 380-389.
[161] Egwurugwu, J.N., C.S. Ufearo, O.C. Abanobi, C.R. Nwokocha, J.O. Duruibe, G.S. Adeleye, A.O. Ebunlomo, A.O. Odetola,and O. Onwufuji (2007) *Afr. J. Biotechnol.* 6 (18): 2078-2082.
[162] Farag, A.G.A., M.E.A. Elhalwagyand H.E. A. Farid (2010) *Pestic. Biochem. Physiology*. 97: 267–274.
[163] Amarnath, R.Y., M. Chalamaiah, B. Ramesh, G. Balaji,and P. Indira (2011) *J. Food Sci. Technol.* 1-7.
[164] Alqasoumi, S., H. Yusufoglu, A. Farraj,and A. Alam (2011) *Int. J. Pharmacol.* 7 (8): 868-873.
[165] Nasri, H., M. Nematbakhsh, S. Ghobadi, R. Ansari, N. Shahinfard,and M. Rafieian-kopaei (2013) *Int. J. Prev. Med.* 4 (3) 316-321.
[166] Mallikarjuna, K., P. SahityaChetan, K. Sathyavelu Reddy,and W. Rajendra (2008) *Fitoterapia.* 79: 174–178.
[167] Shanmugan, K.R., C.H. Ramakrishna, K. Mallikarjuna,and K.Sathyavelu Reddy (2010) *Indian J. Exp. Biol.* 48: 13-149.
[168] Shati, A.A. and F.G. Elsaid (2009) *Food Chem. Toxicol.* 47: 1945–1949.
[169] Bardi, D.A., M.F. Halabi, N.A. Abdullah, E. Rouhollahi, M. Hajrezaie,and M.A. Abdulla (2013) *BioMed. Res. Int.* doi:10.1155/2013/918460.
[170] Weidner, M.S. and K. Sigwart (2000) *J. Ethnopharmacol.* 73: 513–520.
[171] Alnaqeeb, M.A., M. Thomson, K.K. Al-Qattan, F. Kamel, T. Mustafa,and M. Ali (2003) *Kuwait J. Sci. Eng.* 30 (2): 35-48.
[172] Weidner, M.S. and K. Sigwart (2001) *Reprod. Toxicol.* 15: 75–80.
[173] Wilkinson, J.M. (2000) *Reprod. Toxicol.* 14: 507–512.
[174] Dissubandara, D.L.O. and M.S. Chandrasekara (2007) *Ceylon J. Med. Sci.* 50: 1-7.
[175] Jorsarei, S.G.A., Y.R. Yousefnia Pasha, M. Zainalzadeh, A.A. Moghadamnia, A.A. Beiky,and M.R. Damavandi (2008) *Pak. J. Biol. Sci.* 11 (13): 1723-1727.
[176] Nakamura, H. and T. Yamamoto (1983) *Mutat. Res.* 122: 87-94.
[177] Nagabhushan, M., A.J. Amonkarand S.V. Bhide (1986) *Cancer Lett.* 36: 221-233.

[178] Jagetia, G., M. Baligaand P. Venkatesh (2004) *Cancer Biother. Radio.* 19 (4): 422-435.

[179] Shalaby, M.A. and A.R. Hamowieh (2010) *Food Chem. Toxicol.* 48: 2920–2924.

[180] Rong, X., G. Peng, T. Suzuki, Q. Yang, J. Yamahara,and Y. Li (2009) *Regul. Toxicol. Pharm.* 54: 118–123.

[181] Gupta, S., P. Pandotra, A.P. Gupta, J.K. Dhar, G. Sharma, G. Ram, M.K. Husain,and Y.S. Bedi (2010) *Food Chem. Toxicol.* 48: 2966-2971.

In: Ginger
Editor: Janine L. Perry
ISBN: 978-1-63482-020-2

Chapter 2

PHARMACOLOGICAL PROPERTIES AND POTENTIAL ALTERNATIVE USES FOR GINGER (*ZINGIBER OFFICINALE* ROSCOE 1807)

***Karina Zanotti*[1,*] *and Franceli da Silva*[2]**
[1]Nutritionist and PhD in Agricultural Biochemistry. Teacher at the Health Sciences Center, Federal University of Recôncavo da Bahia, Campus Santo Antônio de Jesus, Santo Antônio de Jesus, Bahia, Brazil, CEP
[2]Agronomical Engineer and PhD in Agricultural Engineering, Teacher at the Exact, Environmental and Biological Sciences Center, Federal University of Recôncavo da Bahia, Campus Cruz das Almas, das Almas, Bahia, Brazil, CEP

ABSTRACT

The use of medicinal plants for developing new medications with therapeutic potential deservedly stands out in research. Numerous medicinal species have been reported in the literature, with promising possibilities of discovery of new drugs and also other products, with different potential uses. Ginger (*Zingiber officinale* Roscoe 1807) is of particular interest among these species, since it has been known for millennia and has been widely used by the population, mostly in cookery. Research on the chemical composition of ginger has indicated that it has

* Corresponding author: karinaufrb@ufrb.edu.br.

important biological activity such as antimicrobial and antioxidant action, among other forms of activity. Because of these chemical characteristics, ginger has wide-ranging pharmacological use, with action on metabolism activity and use in treating diseases such as obesity (which is a risk factor for cardiovascular diseases), some types of cancer, psychological disorders and diabetes, among others. Studies have shown the worryingly negative aspects of obesity with regard to the population's health. Thus, adding foods that can enhance metabolic activity, as is the case with ginger, has a direct influence on excessive food intake and constitutes a promising strategy. In addition to characteristics relating to pharmacology, other potential uses broaden the functionality of ginger, such as the fact that this species is considered to be a potential insecticide. Plant extracts from ginger have been used in several types of insect pest control. Moreover, results from research have indicated that ginger can be multifunctional for agriculture, with contributions towards management and control of several food production chains, which broadens the diversity of new products used in agriculture, with the aim of integrated management for agricultural production, thus ensuring food quality. This chapter addresses some interesting aspects of research on the use of ginger for the treating various illnesses and also indicates its potential use in controlling and managing sustainable agricultural production. Ginger is a multifunctional medicinal species, with diverse actions and wide-ranging use for development of new products.

Keywords: Health. *Zingiber officinale* Roscoe. Medicinal plants

1. Introduction

The use of medicinal plants for developing new drugs with therapeutic potential deservedly stands out. Research in this field has indicated that compound extracted from plants present important biological activity (antimicrobial, antioxidant, antitumoral and/or anti-inflammatory activity). Prominent among these is the rhizome of *Zingiber officinale* Roscoe 1807.

Ginger root, the popular name for the rhizome of *Zingiber officinale* Roscoe 1807, is a perennial herbaceous plant that belongs to the *Zingiberaceae* family and originates from the Indo-Malay region. Today, ginger production is widely distributed among the tropical regions of Asia, Africa, Australia and the Americas (YEH et al., 2014).

The *Zingiberaceae* family includes more than 1,200 species distributed among 53 genera, of which the genus *Zingiber* includes some 85 species (Elpo and Negrelle, 2004). The name "Zingiber" for this genus derives from a

Sanskrit word that means "horn-shaped", referring to the bulges on the surface of the rhizome (Steven, 2014).

Taxonomic classification (USDA, 2014):
Kingdom: *Plantae*
Phylum: Magnoliophyta
Class: Liliopsida
Order: Zingiberales
Family: Zingiberaceae
Genus: *Zingiber* p. Moller, 1754
Species: *Zingiber officinale* Roscoe, 1807

India is the largest ginger producer worldwide. Between the years 2009 and 2010, 708,250 tons were produced over an area of 142,090 hectares (Spices Board of India, 2012). This plant's importance in India is not only related to cultural consumption, but also to exportation to Western countries that consume it in significant amounts (Elpo and Negrelle, 2004).

In Brazil, Paraná is the state with the highest production of ginger, totaling 3,945.00 tons/year in an area of 201 hectares distributed among 26 municipalities. The gross annual value of this agricultural production is R$ 3,353,250.19. Ginger ranks third highest in the state of Paraná regarding the production of medicinal, aromatic and condiment plants (Paraná, 2003).

The culinary use of ginger is estimated to have begun more than 2,000 years ago (Bartley and Jacobs, 2000). This root is used for jams, sauces, pickles, drinks and seasoning. Ginger has a striking smell and spicy taste (Jolad et al., 2005), which gives peculiar sensory characteristics to food and has led to consumption almost all over the world (Kubra and Rao, 2012).

Its characteristic aroma and flavor are determined by the composition of its essential oil, which contains sesquiterpene hydrocarbons. Ginger oil has high added value and is exported to the United States and Germany (Spices Board of India, 2012).

A fraction of this oil is used by the pharmaceutical industry for perfumery, while another fraction is used by the food industry, particularly for production of soft drinks (Chari et al., 2012) and additives that give flavor and color to foods (Tilburg et al., 20014).

Ginger is on the American list of additives that are considered safe and do not require new tests, review or clinical trials before its commercialization (http://www.fda.gov/food/IngredientspackagingLabelingGRAS).

The use of ginger in traditional Chinese medicine dates back more than 2,500 years (Braunl and Cohen, 2010). Either raw or processed, it is used as an anti-inflammatory, antiemetic, antitumoral, analgesic and antihemorrhagic agent (Eguchi and Murakami, 2005; RAI et al., 2006), and also as a protector for neuronal cells and an antirheumatic and antifungal agent (Ficker et al., 2003; Sacchetti et al., 2005), and as an antibacterial agent (Sivasothy et al., 2011) and an antiviral agent (Chang et al., 2013). As well as in China, its medicinal use in India, Arabia and Rome was related to the treatment of headaches, colds, fevers and nausea (Ali et al., 2008).

The medicinal use of ginger has motivated many studies over the years. Its benefits towards health are mainly associated with its antioxidant capacity and its chemical components, particularly phenolic substances (Yeh et al., 2014).

The objective of this chapter was to carry out a systematic review of the literature, so as to investigate the pharmacological potential of ginger (*Zingiber officinale* Roscoe).

2. Pharmacological Properties

2.1. Chemical Composition and Antioxidant Activity

Ginger contains more than 400 compounds, including carbohydrates, lipids and polyphenols (Grzanna et al., 2005). Its benefits towards health seem to be related to its total content of phenolic compounds (Yeh et al., 2014).

Polyphenols are the largest group of secondary metabolites in plants. They are present in foods and natural products, and contribute towards their color and flavor. Among the polyphenols that form part of the human diet are phenolic acids, flavonoids, lignin and tannins (polymeric compounds) (Gomes, 2010). The phenolic content of a plant is directly related to its antioxidant capacity (Stefanovits-Banyai et al., 2006).

The main phenolic compound in ginger is 6-gingerol ($C_{17}H_{26}O_4$). It is the main compound responsible for the pungent sensation of ginger and presents high antioxidant capacity (Hessien et al., 2013) (Figure 1).

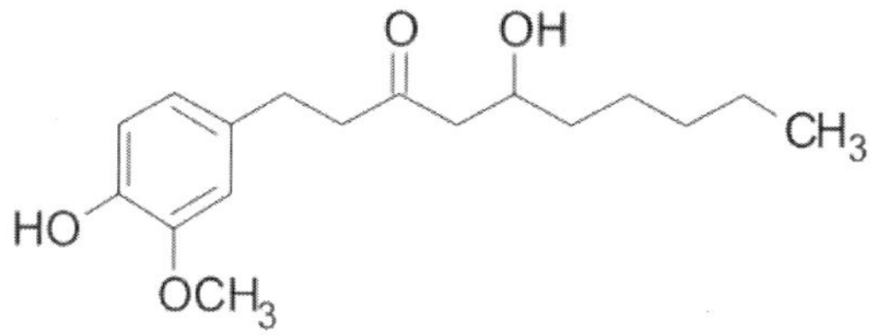

Figure 1. Chemical structure of 6-gingerol (JIN et al., 2014).

Table 1. Gingerol, shogaol and curcumin content in Guangdong ginger and Chu ginger

	Guangdong ginger mg/100 g	Chu ginger mg/100 g
6 -gingerol	5.59 ± 0.09a	4.74 ± 0.11b
6-shogaol	1.41 ± 0.3b	1.85 ± 0.02a
Curcumin	2.32 ± 0.09a	0.96 ± 0.07b

Values expressed as means. Means with different letters differ between each other according to Duncan's test ($p < 0.05$).

Source: Yeh et al., (2014) - adapted.

When gingerols are dehydrated, they are degraded to shogaols and zingerone, which are the main pharmacologically active compounds (Shukla and Singh, 2007). In China, a drug containing 6-shogaol for treating leukemia was patented in 2009 (US20110136916A1; also published as CN101721397A and CN101721397B).

Curcumin, which is another active component of ginger, presents anti-inflammatory activity and high antioxidant, antifungal, antibacterial and antiviral capacity (Motterlini et al., 2000; Joe et al., 2004). Its antioxidant capacity has been shown to be greater than that of vitamin E, which is considered to be a reference antioxidant (Ak and Gulcin, 2008).

Yeh et al. (2014) evaluated two varieties of ginger in Taiwan and demonstrated that the quantities of these compounds differed between the varieties studied (Table 1).

Mezomo et al. (2013) used gas chromatography and identified the following compounds in the essential oil of ginger: α-zingiberene, sesquiphellandrene, farnesene, geranial, bisabolene, curcumene, isobornyl formate, copaene, terpineol, geraniol, pinene, camphene and eucalyptol. These authors also added that these compounds varied in each cultivar, depending on the time of year, type of cultivation, development stage and the vegetative cycle of the plant.

Yeh et al. (2014) identified citric, malic, oxalic, succinic and tartaric acids in ginger, along with 6-shogaol, 6-gingerol, 8-gingerol and 10-gingerol, through high-performance liquid chromatography.

With increasing incidence of non-transmittable chronic diseases, many strategies have been used to control them, acting especially on their risk factors (Fonseca, 2010). One of these strategies has been to investigate natural resources with antioxidant potential.

Antioxidants inhibit reactive oxygen species (Ros), which are capable of causing damage to DNA and are associated with carcinogenesis, coronary disease and many other health issues related to aging (Patel et al., 2000).

Today, natural antioxidants are considered to be important in human diets and in the industry, due to their effects on health. Thus, the demand for them has increase given the growing interest in foods obtained from natural sources (Ibanez et al., 2003).

The antioxidant potential of ginger is associated with its benefits towards health, especially with regard to non-transmittable chronic diseases. A study carried out using ginger demonstrated that its antioxidant activity, according to the Folin-Ciocalteau reagent methodology, was comparable to that of vitamin C, which is another reference antioxidant (Hessien et al., 2013).

A study by Justo et al. (2008) demonstrated that ginger extract from the state of Paraná, Brazil, presented high antioxidant capacity and also a high level of phenolic compounds (136.0 mg GAE/g, i.e. gallic acid equivalent), in comparison with rosemary extract from the same state. In a study by Chanwitheesuk et al. (2005), they showed that the ginger extracts that they used presented 0.601 mg GAE/g, a much lower value than what was found in Paraná.

2.2. Antimicrobial Activity

Natural plant extracts have been used over the years for various purposes, and their potential as drugs and food preservatives has been also been explored (JONES, 1996).

Keeping in mind that food contamination can cause harm to people's health and irreparable loss to the producers of these foods (Zacchino, 2001; Ribeiro et al., 2003; Yahyazadeh et al., 2008), many studies on antimicrobial activity in plant extracts used for preserving raw or processed foods are currently underway, focusing on the antimicrobial compounds in these extracts and their respective mechanisms of action (Lis-Balchin and Deans, 1997).

Studies on the use of antimicrobial agents among humans are expected to show that new drugs derived from plants may have milder collateral effects than those of the current synthetic compounds (Mohanty and Cock, 2009).

Essential oils and plant extracts have been shown to be effective in controlling the growth of various microorganisms, including fungi, bacteria and viruses (Chandarana et al., 2005; Rangel, et al., 2006; Celoto et al., 2008; Roswalka et al., 2008).

At low concentrations, ginger extract has been shown to be effective against human viruses that are responsible for causing respiratory difficulties (Chang et al., 2013).

The methanolic extract of the ginger rhizome was found to be efficient against the bacteria *Escherichia coli*, *Salmonella enteriditis* and *Staphylococcus aureus* (Sunilson et al., 2009).

Gao and Zhang (2010) concluded that ginger extract inhibited the growth of the Gram-positive and Gram-negative bacteria that they analyzed, with no difference between fresh or processed ginger.

Sivasothy et al. (2011) identified bactericidal action from ginger rhizome oil among the following microorganisms: *Bacillus licheniformis*, *Bacillus spizizenii*, *S. aureus*, *E. coli*, *Klebsiella pneumonia* and *Pseudomonas stutzeri*.

2.3. Metabolic Activity

Obesity is one of the risk factors for cardiovascular diseases, some types of cancer, some psychological disorders and diabetes. A large proportion of the population is currently obese and this situation affects all age groups and both sexes and does not depend on economic and social conditions (Pereira et al., 2003). Thus, obesity is considered to be a global epidemic (Popkim and Doak, 1998).

In the light of the significant consequences of obesity towards health, studies have been carried out with a global focus, seeking to identify the main factors that favor its development (Pereira et al., 2003).

Because of the worryingly negative aspects of obesity with regard to health, one promising strategy is to combine foods that can favor metabolic activity, thus directly interfering with excessive consumption of food.

Ginger was used by ancient civilizations (Zich et al., 2008) to treat metabolic illnesses (Schmidt, 2008), especially through the effects demonstrated in peristalsis (O'hara et al., 1998; Afzal et al., 2001), gastric secretions (Nammi et al., 2009) and glucose sensitization (Mansour et al., 2012).

Consumption of powdered ginger leads to decreased lipid peroxidation and lower lipid levels in the plasma and liver of rats treated for eight weeks. Moreover, an increase in the antioxidant capacity of plasma has also been observed (Afshariat, 2007).

Mansour et al. (2012) observed that consumption of ginger causes thermogenesis and can decrease the feeling of hunger, thus potentially leading to lower food consumption. These authors concluded that ginger presents properties that control body weight, in their study carried out among obese men.

A study on rats fed on a diet rich in lipids and ginger for six weeks demonstrated that these animals presented lower weight gain, and lower levels of insulin, glucose, total cholesterol, LDL, VLDL, free fatty acids, phospholipids and triglycerides, in comparison with animals that received the same diet rich in lipids but without ginger (Nammi et al., 2009).

Use of powdered ginger dissolved in warm water was able to modulate the appetite of obese men, through increasing satiety, gastric plenitude and reducing hunger (Mansour et al., 2012).

Atashak et al. (2014) suggested that obese patients undergoing resistance training should consume ginger to aid in their antioxidant processes, since ginger has been shown to be effective in increasing antioxidant activity in plasma.

From a public health point of view, Mansour et al. (2012) suggested that because ginger produces an increased thermal effect and greater satiety, without adverse undesirable effects, its use may be important for weight control treatment.

Regarding obesity, all strategies and initiatives that suggest beneficial effects should be encouraged and studied in detail, so as to provide support for possible treatment options.

2.4. Antiemetic and Anti-Nausea Activity during Pregnancy

One of the most common and uncomfortable complications of pregnancy is nausea and vomiting. Some women progress badly and require medical assistance to treat these ailments during pregnancy. Between 50 and 80% of pregnant women report that they are affected by vomiting and nausea, especially during the first trimester of gestation (Fisher-Rasmussen et al., 1991).

The use of medication to relieve symptoms is often contraindicated. However, many medicinal plants are used in alternative medicine, and ginger is among them (Blumenthal, 2000).

Ginger is used against vomiting and nausea in traditional Chinese medicine (Wichtl, 2004) and its mechanism of action seems to be associated with increased gastric tonus and peristalsis, through anticholinergic and antiserotonergic pathways (Wilkinson, 2000).

Regarding safe use of ginger during pregnancy, exposure to this plant does not seem to increase the risk of fetal malformations, low weight at birth, prenatal hemorrhage, postpartum hemorrhage (Willetts et al., 2003), fetal complications or abnormalities (Keating and Chez, 2002) among women treated with ginger.

Regarding the efficacy of administering ginger for nausea and vomiting among pregnant women, a study by Keating and Chez (2002) demonstrated that administering 250 mg of ginger for two weeks gave rise to less feeling of nausea and vomiting among the treated pregnant women, in comparison with a placebo group.

Ozgoli et al. (2009) administered 250 mg of ginger for four days and observed that ginger was significantly more effective than placebo in reducing the frequency of vomiting and the intensity of nausea ($p < 0.05$). This treatment did not present side effects.

Smith et al. (2004) administered a higher dose (350 mg) for three weeks and concluded that ginger was as effective against nausea and vomiting as vitamin B6, a drug that is used for the same purpose.

Willetts et al. (2003) used the equivalent of 1.5 g of dry ginger for four days and obtained the result that ginger was significantly more effective than placebo for the reported nausea, but not for the vomiting.

Ding et al. (2013) indicated that ginger treatment may be effective during pregnancy against nausea and vomiting. However, these authors did not find evidence in the studies evaluated in their review article regarding the maximum safe dosage, treatment period or consequences from overdoses. High doses could aggravate preexisting conditions such as cholelithiasis (Hardy and Udani, 2004) and could contribute towards heart arrhythmia and cause heartburn (Westfall, 2004).

2.5. Antidiabetic Action

Diabetes mellitus is a disease characterized by high levels of glucose in the patient's blood. These high levels may occur due to absence of insulin production or inefficient production, or even both factors. It has been estimated that by 2030, more than 366 million people will have diabetes mellitus (Rathmann and Giani, 2004).

Chinese medicine has been using ginger as a hypoglycemic substance for centuries. It is believed that ginger inhibits hepatic phosphorylase, thereby reducing hepatic glycogenolysis and increasing the activity of enzymes responsible for glycogenesis, as well as inhibiting glucose-6-phosphatase, thus reducing glucose (Zhang and Tan, 2000).

In a study carried out by Shirdel et al. (2009), the antidiabetic effect of ginger was tested among diabetic mice. The results showed that there was a significant reduction in the serum glucose of these animals.

Goyal et al. (2006), in India, observed a significant decrease in glucose among diabetic mice treated with ginger. The same result was also observed by Singh et al. (2009) in India.

Al-Amin et al. (2006) indicated that the aqueous extract of fresh ginger administered every day (500 mg/kg, intraperitoneally) to diabetic rats, over a seven-week period, presented a hypoglycemic effect.

Mozaffari-Khosravi et al. (2014) indicated that daily consumption of 3 g of powdered ginger by patients with type 2 diabetes over an eight-week period caused an improvement in glycemic indices and insulin resistance. This study's limitation was the short treatment period, and the authors also reported that studies on the adverse effects of ginger should also be conducted.

Diabetes mellitus is a risk factor in many other diseases that affect thousands of people all over the world. Measures that can control it will directly influence the quality of life of these people and public health factors.

3. Potential Other Uses for Ginger

The Zingiberaceae family is distributed in tropical and semitropical areas, including 50 genera and 1,100 species. From an economic point of view, *Zingiber officinale* Roscoe is of particular interest, with its aromatic rhizomes (Souza, 2005; Dabague, 2008).

Ginger is an erect, rhizomatous plant, of approximately 50 cm in height, with lance-shaped simple leaves of 15-30 cm in length. The flowers are sterile and white-yellow in color. The rhizome is jointed, septate and fleshy, covered by a rough skin, from which the aerial stem develops. In its lower portion, the plant presents many cylindrical rhizomes that are horizontal, laterally distributed and fingerlike, with ramifications in the same plane, and which present scars at their apex due to the foliaceous stems, measuring 14 to 16 cm in length by 4 to 20 mm in width (Lorenzi and Matos, 2008).

Essential ginger oil is slightly yellow and fluid, with an oily appearance at room temperature. It consists mainly of monoterpenes and sesquiterpenes (Sacchetti et al., 2004).

The use of ginger (*Zingiber officinale* Roscoe; Zingiberaceae) is widely known in cooking as a seasoning, but the Chinese have also used it in medicine for a very long time (Sabulal et al., 2006).

Campanhola and Bettiol (2003) reported that one way to decrease the intensive use of pesticides in the environment is by using alternative phytosanitary control measures, such as the use of plant extracts and hydrolates. Ginger is a multifunctional plant, with properties that qualify it as having potential use as an insecticide plant.

Although pesticides have contributed towards food production, their indiscriminate use over a prolonged period has caused negative impacts on human health and changes to the production environment. Products derived from insecticide plants are of interest for pest insect control because they offer lower risk to human and animal health. Thus, these have been the target of several research efforts (Silva et al., 2013).

According to Silva (2009), ginger extracts are widely used in phytopathogen control. Rozwalka et al. (2008) reported that ginger extract presented an inhibitory effect towards *Colletotrichum gloeosporioides* regarding mycelial growth.

The effect of crude *Z. officinale* extract, incorporated into potato dextrose agar (PDA) culture medium at concentrations of 1, 5, 10, 15, 20, 25 and 50%, was studied regarding the mycelial growth of *Alternaria solani* (Ell. and Mart.) Jones and Grout, *A. alternata* (Fr.) Kiessler, *Sclerotium rolfsii* Sacc., *Rhizoctonia solani* Kühn and *Colletotrichum graminicola* (Ces.) G.W. Wils. That study showed 100% inhibition of mycelial growth for *C. graminicola, R. solani, S. rolfsii* and *C. graminicola* at concentrations of 5%, 50%, 20% and 10% of the extract, respectively (Rodrigues et al., 1999).

Plant extracts with insecticide activity act as tools for management and control of pest insects, especially in small farming areas. Thus, they contributing towards food safety and decreasing the impact of pesticides on the environment, as well as acting as the basis for strengthening the principles of agroecology (Dequech, 2008; Silva, 2009).

However, these products also present disadvantages such as toxicity to beneficial insects and low persistency. Some of them are toxic to mammals and fish, and the active agents of the plants fluctuate according to the management used in their production and the edaphoclimatic factors of the region from which they are harvested (Roel, 2001; Corrêa; Salgado, 2011). Nevertheless, taking the interactions with the environment into account, these plant extracts demonstrate potential for the discovery of new products, with the aim of integrated management of agricultural production and assured quality for the food produced.

Berlitz and Fiuza (2004) reported that ginger extracts added to artificial diets and offered to second-instar *A. gemmtalis* caterpillars presented a cytotoxic effect, through presenting epithelial disruption 48 hours after the treatments were applied.

Silva (2009) used aqueous extracts of ginger at dosages of 0.7, 0.8 and 0.9 g/mL to control *Toxoptera citricida* Kirk., 1907 (Hemiptera: Aphididae) and concluded that 24 hours after application, these dosages presented control potential such that the survival rates were 22%, 30% and 30%, respectively. After 48 hours, the survival rates decreased to 8%, 7% and 3%, thus demonstrating the potential use of these extracts for pest-insect control.

In Brazil, ginger extract has been tested and researched due to its insecticide potential for control and management of the white fly (*Aleurothrixus aepim* (Goeldi), 1886 (Hemiptera: Aleyrodidae), in cassava (manioc) crops (*Manihot esculenta* Crantz).

Cassava (*Manihot esculenta* Crantz) originated from South America, where it was domesticated for root production (Fukuda; Iglesias, 2006). This plant can be found in several ecological regions, thus demonstrating its adaptability to different climatic regions (Oliveira et al., 2006). Cassava is one of the main sources of carbohydrates in the tropics (Souza et al., 2006). In addition to its use in agriculture, as a form of subsistence crop, cassava has had an important role in the food, paper and textile industries for the preparation of pigments and for fabric finishing (Sebrae, 2008). Because cassava has a long growth cycle, it provides favorable conditions for attack by several arthropods, especially the white fly *Aleurothrixus aepim* (Goeldi, 1886) (Hemiptera: Aleyrodidae) (Farias; Bellotti, 2006). The white fly is important not only because this is a pest insect of agricultural interest, but also because the species may be a vector for viral diseases (Moreno, 2002). According to Oliveira and Lima (2006), the greatest threat to cassava cultivation in Africa comes from the white fly *Bemisia tabaci* (Gennadius, 1889), which causes serious damage to production, through transmission of the African cassava mosaic virus (ACMV).

Neem (*Azadirachta indica* A.) (Lima et al., 2011), epazote (*Chenopodium ambrosioides* L.) (Mazzonetto; Vendramim, 2003) and ginger (*Zingiber officinale* Roscoe) (Silva, 2009) are among the plants with potential for controlling the white fly in cassava.

Silva (2013) evaluated the toxicity of aqueous extracts of insecticide plants and commercial neem-based products on the incidence of white flies (*Aleurothrixus aepim* (Goeldi), 1886) (Hemiptera: Aleyrodidae), at different concentrations of white fly eggs and nymphs in cassava crops (*Manihot esculenta* Crantz). This author observed that extracts of *Z. officinale* (70%), *A. indica* seeds (7.9%), Organic Neem® (0.75%) and Azamax® (0.25%) decreased survival after the third application. The commercial product Azamax® (0.50%) caused 100% mortality among white fly nymphs, eleven days after the first application. *C. ambrosioides* extracts at concentrations of 60 and 70% caused the greatest mortality among white fly eggs. *Z. officinale* extracts (60%), Organic Neem® (0.75%) and Azamax® (0.50%) affected the development of white fly nymphs. Thus, the study demonstrated that ginger presents insecticide potential and that its chemical composition can be used in the future to originate commercial products.

Studies on the potential use of ginger need to be improved not only within the field of healthcare, but also in relation to development of its production chain. These improvements should aim towards discovery of new products and processes that can contribute in the future to the development of sustainable agriculture and higher-quality products for the population.

FINAL REMARKS

Ginger presents high pharmacological potential and alternative uses, especially regarding its antioxidant capacity, which is directly related to controlling non-transmittable chronic diseases. The studies mentioned here indicate that research should be intensified regarding the use of ginger for treating several illnesses and also for broadening its use in controlling and managing sustainable agricultural production. Ginger has pharmacological potential and also potential use in agroecosystems in the form of products, for control and management purposes in areas of agricultural production.

REFERENCES

Afshari AT, A. T., Shirpoor, A., Farshid, A., Saadatian, R., Rasmi, Y., Saboory, E., Ilkhanizadeh, B. & Allameh, A. (2007). The effect of ginger on diabetic nephropathy, plasma antioxidant capacity and lipid peroxidation in rats. *Food Chem. 10*, 148-153.

Afzal, M., Al-Hadidi, D., Menon, M., Pesek, J. & Dhami, M. S. (2001). Ginger: an ethnomedical, chemical and pharmacological review. *Drug Metabol Drug Interact*, *18*,159–190.

AK, T. & Gulcin, I. (2008). Antioxidant and radical scavenging properties of curcumin. *Chemico-Biological Interactions*, *174*, 27-37.

Al-Amin, Z. M., Thomson, M., Al-Qattan, K. K., Peltonen-Shalaby, R. & Ali, M. (2006). Anti-diabetic and hypolipidaemic properties of ginger (*Zingiber officinale*) in streptozotocin-induced diabetic rats. *Br J Nutr*, *96*, 4, 660-666.

Ali, B. H., Blunden, G., Tanira, M. O. & Nemmar, A. (2008). Some phytochemical, pharmacological and toxicological properties of ginger (*Zingiber officinale* Roscoe): A review of recent research. *Food and Chemical Toxicology*, *46*, 409-420.

Atashak, S., Peeri, M., Azarbayjani, A. M. & Stannard, S. R. (2014). Effects of ginger (*Zingiber officinale* Roscoe) supplementation and resistance training on some blood oxidative stress markers in obese men *Journal of Exercise Science & Fitness*, *12*, 26-30.

Bartley, J. & E Jacobs, A. (2000). Effects of drying on flavour compounds in Australian grown ginger (*Zingiber officinale*). *Journal of the Science of Food and Agriculture*, *80*, 209-215.

Berlitz, D. L. & E Fiuza, L. M. (2004). Avaliação toxicológica de *Bacillus thuringiensis aizawai* para *Spodoptera frugipera* (Lepidoptera: Noctuidae), *Em Laboratório. Biociências*, *12*(2), 115-119p.

Blumenthal, M. (2000). Expanded commission e monographs. Boston: Integrative Medicine Publications.

Braun, L., Cohen, M. (2010). Herbs & Natural Supplements. 3rd ed. Sydney, Australia: Churchill Livingstone.

Campanhola, C. & Bettiol, W. (2003). Métodos alternativos de controle fitossanitário. Jaguariúna: Embrapa Meio Ambiente, 279p.

Chandarana, H., Baluja, S. & Chanda, S. V. (2005). Comparison of antibacterial activities of selected species of Zingiberaceae family and some synthetic compounds, *Turkish Journal of Biology*, *29*, 83-97.

Chanwitheesuk, A., Theerawutgulung, A. & Rakhariyatham, N. (2005). Screening of antioxidant activity and antioxidant compounds of some edible plants of Thailand. *Food Chem*, *92*, 491.

Celoto, M. I. B., Papa, M. F. S., Sacramento, L. V. S. & Celoto, F. J. (2008). Atividade antifúngica de extratos de plantas a Colletotrichum gloeosporioides. *Acta Scientiarum*, *30*, 1, 1-5.

Chang, J. S., Wanga, K. C., Yeh, C. F., Shieh, D. E. & Chiang, L. C. (2013). Fresh ginger (*Zingiber officinale*) hasanti-viral activity against human respiratory syncytial virus in human respiratory tractcelllines *Journal of Ethnopharmacology*, *145*, 146-151.

Chari, N. K. L., Manasa, D., Srinivas, P. & Sowbhagya, H. B. (2013). Enzyme-assisted extraction of bioactive compounds from ginger (*Zingiber officinale* Roscoe), *Food Chemistry*, *139*, 509-514.

Conselho De Especiarias Da India, Spices Board, Kochi, India. (2012).

Corrêa, J. C. R. & Salgado, H. R. N. (2011). Atividade inseticida das plantas e aplicações: revisão. *Revista Brasileira de Plantas Medicinais, Botucatu*, *13*, 4, 500-506,

Ding, M., Leach, M. & Bradley, H. (2013). The effectiveness and safety of ginger for pregnancy-induced nausea and vomiting: *A systematic review Women and Birth*, *26*, 26-30.

Dequech, S. T. B. (2008). et al. Fitotoxicidade causada por inseticidas botânicos em feijão-de-vagem (*Phaseolus vulgaris* L.) cultivado em estufa plástica. Revista da Faculdade de Zootecnia, Veterinária e Agronomia. v. 15, n.1, pag. 71-80.

Eguchi, A., Murakami, H. & Ohigashi, A. (2005). Novel bioassay system for evaluating anti-oxidative activities of food items: use of basolateral media from differentiated Caco-e cells, *Free Radical Research*, *39*, 1367-1375.

Elpo, E. R. S. & Negrelle, R. R. B. (2004). *Zingiber officinale* ROSCOE: Aspectos Botânicos E Ecológicos. Visão Acadêmica, *Curitiba*, *5*, 1, 27-32.

Farias, A. R. N. & Bellotti, A. C. (2006). Pragas e seu controle. In.: SOUZA, L. da S. et al. (Ed.). Aspectos socioeconômicos e agronômicos da mandioca. Cruz das Almas: Embrapa Mandioca e Fruticultura, *Cap. 20*, 591-691.

Ficker, C., Smith, M. L., Akpagana, K., Gbeassor, M., Zhang, J., Durst, T., Assabgui, R. & Arnason, J. T. (2003). Bioassay-guided isolation and identification of antifungal com-pounds from ginger, *Phytotherapy Research*, *17*, 897-902.

Fisher-Rasmussen, W., Kjaer, S. K. & Dahl, C. (1991). Ginger treatment of hyperemesis gravidarum. *European Journal of Obstetrics Gynecology and Reproductive Biology*, *42*, 163-164.

Fonseca, K. Z. (2010). Ação do resveratrol e das tinturas das cascas e das folhas de *Vitis labrusca* L. var. *Isabel* na hiperlipidemia induzida em coelhos. / Dissertação de Mestrado, UFOP, Ouro Preto.

Fukuda, W. M. G. & Iglesias, C. (2006). Recursos genéticos. In: Souza, L. da S. et al. (Ed.). Aspectos socioeconômicos e agronômicos da mandioca. Cruz das Almas: Embrapa Mandioca e Fruticultura Tropical, *Cap. 12*, p.301-323.

Gao, D. & Zhang, Y. (2010). Comparative antibacterial activities of extracts of dried ginger and processed ginger. *Pharmacognosy Journal*, *2*, 41-44.

Gomes, S. M. C. (2010). Determinação de antioxidantes por cromatografia líquida de alta pressão com detecção electroquímica. Dissertação de mestrado. Coimbra.

Goyal, R. K. & Kadnur, S. V. (2006). Beneficial effects of *Zingiber officinale* on goldthio glucose induced obesity. *Fitoterapia*, *77*, 3, 160-163.

Gras. F. D. A. (http://www.fda.gov/Food/IngredientsPackagingLabeling/ GRAS / ucm2006850.htm).

Grzanna R., Lindmark, L. & Frondoza, C. G. (2005). Ginger-an herbal medicinal product with broad anti-inflammatory actions. *Journal of Medicinal Food*, *8*, 2, 125-32.

Hardy, M. & Udani, J. (2004). Does ginger help with symptoms of nausea in early pregnancy? *Alternative Therapies in Women's Health*, *6*, 25-29.

Ibañez, E., Kubátová, A., Señorans, F. J., Cavero, S., Reglero, G. & Hawthorne, S. B. (2003). Subcritical water extraction of antioxidant compounds from rosemary plants. *Journal of Agricultural and Food Chemistry*, *51*, 375-382.

Jin, Z., Lee, G., Kim, S., Park, C. S., Park, Y. S. & Jin, Y. H. (2014). Ginger and Its Pungent Constituents Non-Competitively Inhibit Serotonin Currents on Visceral Afferent Neurons. *Korean J Physiol Pharmacol.* 18, 2, 149-153.

Joe, B., Vijaykumar, M. & Lokesh, B. R. (2004). Biological properties of curcumin cellular and molecular mechanisms of action. *Critical Reviews in Food Science and Nutrition*, *44*, 97-111.

Jolad, S. D., Lantz, R. C., Chen, G. J., Bates, R. B. & Timmermann, B. N. (2005). Commercially processed dry ginger (*Zingiber officinale*): Composition and effects on LPS-stimulated PGE2 production. *Phytochemistry*, *66*, 1614-1635.

Jones, F. A. (1996). Herbs – useful plants. Their role in history and today, *European Journal Gastroenterology & Hepatology*, *8*, 1227-1231.

Keating, A. & Chez, R. (2002). Ginger syrup as an antiemetic in early pregnancy. *Alternative Therapies in Health and Medicine*, *8*, 89-91.

Kubra, I. R. & E Rao, L. J. M. (2012). An impression on current developments in the technology, chemistry, and biological activities of ginger (*Zingiber officinale* Roscoe). *Critical Reviews in Food Science and Nutrition*, *52*(8), 651-688.

Li, P., Peng Y., Lianwen, Q., Wen, X., Ma, J., Zhou, P., Zhang, L., Liu, Q., Liu, E. & Chen, J. (2011). inventores. 6-shogaol for using in a method for the treatment of leukemia.Estados Unidos, patente US n. US 12/938,949, 2009 Dez 8, Jun 9.

Lis-Balchin, M. & Deans, S. G. (1997). Bioactivity of selected plant essential oils againstListeria monocytogenes, *Journal of Applied Bacteriology*, *82*, 759-762.

Lima, B. M. F. V., Moreira, J. O. T. & Pinto, H. C. S. (2011). Avaliação de extratos vegetais no controle de mosca-branca em tomate. *Revista Caatinga, Mossoró-RN*, v. *24*. 4, 36-42,

Lorenzi, H. & Matos, F. J. A. (2008). Plantas medicinais do Brasil: nativas e exóticas. 2ª. ed. Nova Odessa, SP: Plantarum, 544.

Paraná. Secretaria Municipal do Abastecimento de Curitiba. Divisão de conjuntura econômica e controle estatístico. Dados obtidos da comercialização de gengibre. Curitiba, PR, (2002).

Patel, R. P., Moellering, D., Murphy-Ullrich, J., Jo, H., Beckman, J. S. & Darley-Usmar, V. M. (2000). Cell signaling by reactive nitrogen and oxygen species in atherosclerosis. *Free Radical Biology*, *28*, 1780-1794.

Pereira, I. O., Francischi, R. P. & Lancha Jr, A. H. (2003). Obesidade: Hábitos Nutricionais, Sedentarismo e Resistência à Insulina. *Arq Bras Endocrinol Metab*, *47*, 2, 111-127.

Popkin, B. M. & Doak, C. M. (1998). The obesity epidemic is a worldwide phenomenon. *Nutr Rev*, *56*, 106-114.

Mesomo, M. C., Corazza, M. L., Ndiayea, P. M., Osmar, R., Santab, D., Cardozo, L. & Scheera, A. P. (2013). Supercritical CO2 extracts and essential oil of ginger (*Zingiber officinale* R.): Chemical composition and antibacterial activity. *Supercritical Fluids*, *80*, 44-49,

Miranda, A. L., Tilburg, V., Olafur, S., Palsson, Y. & Ringel, W. (2014). E. Is ginger effective for the treatment of irritable bowel syndrome? A double blind randomized controlled pilot trial. *Whitehead Complementary Therapies in Medicine*, *22*, 17-20.

Moreno, L. L. V. (2002). Avances del control biologico de *Bemisia tabaci* en la region neotropical. Manejo Integrado de Plagas y Agroecología, Costa Rica, n. *66*, p. 82-95.

Mazzonetto, F. & Vendramim, J. D. (2003). Efeito de pós de origem vegetal sobre *Acanthoscelides obtectus* (Say) (Coleoptera: Bruchidae) em feijão armazenado. *Neotropical Entomology*, v. *32*, 145-149.

Mohanty, S. & Cock, I. E. (2009). Evaluation of the antibacterial activity and toxicity of *Myrciaria caulifloria* methanolic leaf and fruit extracts, *Internet Journal of Microbiology*, *7* (Suppl. 2).

Mohamed, H. T., Horia, D., Saad, E. G. & Morsy, A. S. (2013). Unfractionated green tea and ginger polyphenols induce apoptotic, cytotoxic and antioxidant effects in hepatoma cells. *Journal of herbal medicine*. 387-398.

Motterlini, R., Foresti, R., Bassi, R. & Green, C. J. (2000). Curcumin, an antioxidant and anti-inflammatory agent, induces heme oxygenase-1 and protects endothelial cells against oxidative stress. *Free Radical Biology and Medicine*, *28*, 1303-1312.

Mozaffari-Khosravi, H., Talaei, B., Jalali, B. A., Najarzadeh, A., Mozayan, M. R. (2014). The effect of ginger powder supplementation on insulin resistance and glycemic indices in patients with type 2 diabetes: a randomized, double-blind, placebo-controlled trial. Complement *Ther Med*. *22*, 1, 9-16.

Muhammad, S., Mansoura, Y. M. N., Amy, L., Roberts, M. K., Arindam, R. & Choudhuryc, M. P. S. (2012). Ginger consumption enhances the thermic effect of food and promotes feelings of satiety without affecting metabolic and hormonal parameters in overweight men: *A pilot study metabolism clinical and experimental*, *61*, 1347-1352.

Nammi, S., Sreemantula, S. & Roufogalis, B. D. (2009). Protective effects of ethanolic extract of Zingiber officinale rhizome on the development of metabolic syndrome in high-fat diet-fed rats. *Basic Clin Pharmacol Toxicol*, *104*, 366–373.

O'hara, M., Kiefer, D., Farrell, K. & Kemper, K. (1998). A review of 12 commonly used medicinal herbs. *Archives of Family Medicine*, *7*, 523-536.

Ozgoli, G., Goli, M. & Simbar, M. (2009). Effects of ginger capsules on pregnancy, nausea, and vomiting. *Journal of Alternative and Complementary Medicine*, *15*, 243-246.

Oliveira, S. L., Coelho, E. F., Nogueira, C. C. P., Irrigação. In: SOUZA, L. da S. et al. (Ed.). Aspectos socioeconômicos e agronômicos da mandioca.

Cruz das Almas: Embrapa Mandioca e Fruticultura Tropical, 2006. *Cap.11*, p.291-300.

Oliveira, M. R. V. & Lima, L. H. C. (2006). Moscas-brancas na cultura da mandioca no Brasil. Brasília-DF: Embrapa Recursos Genéticos e Biotecnologia,_74.p. (Documentos 186).

Rai, S., Mukherjee, K., Mal, M., Wahile, A., Saha, B. P. & Mukherjee, P. K. (2006). Determination of 6-gingerol in ginger (*Zingiber officinale*) using high-performance thin-layerchromatography, *Journal of Separation Science*, *29*, 2292-2295.

Rangel, M. A. S., Gabriel, M. & Smiderle, O. J. (2006). Avaliação de substâncias alternativas para proteção de grãos de soja contra fungos. In: III CONGRESSO BRASILEIRO DE DEFENSIVOS AGRÍCOLAS *NATURAIS*, *3*, 2006, Belém. Anais...Belém-PA,

Rathmann W. & Giani G. (2004). Global prevalence of diabetes: estimates for the year 2000 and projections for 2030. *Diabetes Care*, *27*, 10, 2568-2569.

Ribeiro, S. A., Cavalcanti, M. A., Fernandes, M. J. & Lima, D. M. (2003). Fungos filamentosos isolados de produtos derivados do milho comercializados em Recife, *Pernambuco. Revista Brasileira de Botânica*, *26*, 2, 223-229,

Rozwalka, L. C., Lima, M. L. R. Z. C., Mio, L. L. M. & Nakashima, T. (2008). Extratos, decoctos e óleos essenciais de plantas medicinais e aromáticas na inibição de *Glomerella cingulata* e *Colletotrichum gloeosporioides* de frutos de goiaba. *Ciência rural*, *38*, 2, 301- 307.

Roel, A. R. (2001). Uso de plantas com propriedades inseticidas: uma contribuição para o desenvolvimento rural sustentável. Revista Internacional de Desenvolvimento Local, *Campo Grande*, *MS*, v. *1*, n. 2, p. 43-50.

Rodrigues, B. N., Passini, T. & Ferreira, A. G. (1999). Research on allelopathy in Brazil. In: NARWAL, S.S. (Ed.) Allelopathy Update Enfield, *Science Pub.*, *1*, 307-323.

Sacchetti, G., Maietti, S., Muzzoli, M., Scaglianti, M., Manfredini, S. & Radice, M. (2005). Comparative evaluation off 11 essential oils of different origin as functional antioxidants, antiradicals and antimicrobials in food, *Food Chemistry*, *91* (Suppl.4) 621–632.

Sacchetti, G., Medici, A., Maietti, S., Radice,M., Muzzoli, M., Manfredini, S., Braccioli, E. & Bruni R. (2004). Composition and Functional Properties of the Essential Oil of Amazonian Basil, *Ocimum micranthum* Willd., Labiatae in Comparison with Commercial Essential Oils. *Journal of Agricultural and Food Chemistry*, v. *52*, n. 11, p. 3486-3491,

Sabulal, B., Dan, M., J. A. J., Kurup, R., Pradeep, N. S., Valsamma, R. K., George, V. (2006). Caruophyllene-rich rhizome oil of *Zingiber nimmonni* from South India: Chemical characterization and antimicrobial activity. *Phytochemistry*, *67*, 2469-2473.

Sebrae. (2008). Estudo de mercado sobre a mandioca. Relatório completo.

Schmidt, B., Ribnicky, D. M., Poulev, A., Logendra, S., Cefalu, W. T., Raskin, I. (2008). *A natural history of botanical therapeutics.Metabolism*, *57*, 3-9.

Shirdel, Z., Mirbadalzadeh, H. & Madani, H. (2009). Anti-diabetic and anti lipidemic properties of ginger in comparison glibenclamide in alloxan-diabetes rat. *Iran J Diab Lipid Disorders*, *9*, 1, 7-15.

Shukla, Y., Singh, M. (2007). Cancer preventive properties of ginger: a brief review. *Food and Chemical Toxicology*, *45*, 5, 683-90.

Singh, A., Akanksha Singh, N., Maurya, R. & Arvind Kumar, S. (2009). Anti-hyperglycaemic, lipid lowering and anti-oxidant properties of 6-gingerol in db/db mice. *Int J Med Sci*, *1*, 12, 536-544.

Sivasothy, Y., Chong, W. K., Hamid, A., Eldeen, I. M., Sulaiman, S. F. & Awang, K. (2011). Essential oils of *Zingiber officinale* var. *rubrum* Theilade and their antibacterialactivities, *Food Chemistry*, *124*, 514-517.

Silva, M. P. L. (2009). Bioatividade de extratos vegetais no controle de pulgão preto Toxoptera citricida Kirk.,1907 (Hemiptera: Aphididae) na cultura dos citros e sobrevivência de joaninhas e abelhas. 79f. Dissertação (Mestrado) - UFRB, Cruz das Almas-BA.

Silva, M. P. L. et al., (2009). Atividade inseticida de Extrato Aquoso de Gengibre *Zingiber officinale* L. no Controle do Pulgão preto *Toxoptera citricida* (Kirkaldy) (Hemíptera: Aphididae) em Citros. *Revista Brasileira de Agroecologia*, v.*4*, n. 2, p. 677-680, nov.

Silva, M. P. L. (2013). Avaliação do potencial de plantas inseticidas no controle de *Aleurothrixus aepim* Goeldi, 1886 (Hemiptera: Aleyrodidae) em mandioca *Manihot esculenta* Crantz. Tese de Doutorado. Cruz das Almas, BA.

Smith, C., Crowther, C., Willson, K., Hotham, N. & Mcmilliam, V. A. (2004). randomized controlled trial of ginger to treat nausea and vomiting in pregnancy. *Obstetrics and Gynecology*, *103*, 639-645.

Stefanovits-Banyai, E., Szentrnihalyi, K., Hegedüs, A., Koczka, N., Vali, L., Taba, G. & Blazovics, A. (2006). Metal ion and antioxidant alterations in leaves between different sexes of *Ginkgo biloba L. Life Sci.*, *78*, 1049.

Stevem Foster Group, Inc. Ginger *Zingiber Officinale* — Your Food Is Your Medicine**.** Disponível em: < http://www. stevenfoster. com/education/ monograph /ginger. html >. Acesso em: 04/09/2014.

Souza, A. P. & Vendramim, J. D. (2005). Efeito translaminar, sistêmico e de contato de extrato aquoso de sementes de nim sobre *Bemisia tabaci* (Genn.) Biótipo B em tomateiro. *Neotropical Entomology*, *34*, 1, 83-87.

Sunilson, J. A. J., Suraj, R., Rejitha, G. & Anandarajagopa, K. (2009). In vitro antibacte-rial evaluation of *Zingiber officinale*, Curcuma longa and Alpinia galangal extractsas natural foods preservatives, *American Journal of Food Technology*, *4*, 192–200.

United States Department of Agriculture. Natural Resources Conservation Service: Classification. Disponível em: http://plants.usda.gov/core/profile?symbol=ZIOF. Acesso em: 04/09/2014.

Westfall, R. (2004). Use of antiemetic herbs in pregnancy: women's choices, and the question of safety and efficacy. *Complementary Therapies in Nursing and Midwifery*, *10*, 30-36.

Wichtl, M. (2004). Herbal drugs and phytopharmaceuticals. 3rd ed. Boca Raton, Florida:CRC Press.

Wilkinson J. (2000). What do we know about herbal morning sickness treatments? A literature survey. *Midwifery*, *16*, 224-228.

Willetts, K., Ekangaki, A. & Eden, J. (2003). Effect of a ginger extract on pregnancy-induced nausea: a randomised controlled trial. *Australian & New Zealand Journal of Obstretics & Gynaecology*, *43*, 139-144.

Zacchino, S. (2001). Estratégia para a descoberta de novos agentes antifúngicos. In: YUNES, R.A. E CALIXTO, J.B. Plantas medicinais sob a ótica da química medicinal moderna. *Argos*, 435-479.

Zhang, X. F. & Tan, B. K. (2000). Effects of an ethanolic extract of *Gynura procumbens* on serum glucose, cholesterol and triglyceride levels in normal and streptozotocin-induced diabetic rats. *Singapore Med J*, *41*, 1, 9-13.

Zick Sm, Djuric, Z., Ruffin, M. T., Litzinger, A. J., Normolle, D. P., Alrawi, S. Feng, M. R. & Brenner, D. E. (2008). Pharmacokinetics of 6-gingerol, 8-gingerol, 10-gingerol, and 6-shogaol and conjugate metabolites in healthy human subjects. *Cancer Epidemiol Biomarkers Prev*, *17*, 1930-1936.

Yahyazadeh, M., Omidbaigi, R., Zare, R., Taheri, H. (2008). Effect of some essential oils on mycelial growth of *Penicillium digitatum Sacc*. World *Journal of Microbiology and Biotechnology*, *24*, 1445-1450.

Yeh, H. Y., Chuang, C. H., Chen, H. C., Wan, C. J., Chean, T. L., Lin, L. Y. (2014). Bioactive components analysis of two various gingers (*Zingiber officinale* Roscoe) and antioxidant effect of ginger extracts. *LWT - Food Science and Technology*, *55*, 329-334.

In: Ginger
Editor: Janine L. Perry
ISBN: 978-1-63482-020-2

Chapter 3

ANTIOXIDANT ACTIVITY OF GINGER

Tzi Bun Ng* and Charlene Cheuk Wing Ng
School of Biomedical Sciences, Faculty of Medicine,
The Chinese University of Hong Kong,
New Territories, Hong Kong, China

ABSTRACT

The rhizome, stem and leaves of ginger (*Zingiber officinale*) exhibit antioxidant activity. However, the bulk of studies was done using the rhizome extract and some were performed using the essential oil. Compounds have been isolated and chemically characterized from ginger. The anti-diabetic, neuroprotective, gastroprotective, nephroprotective, and cardioprotective actions of ginger are related to its antioxidant activity. Ginger has a beneficial effect on male reproduction in rodents and broiler chickens. It ameliorates the toxicity of insecticides. These actions may also be related to its antioxidant activity.

INTRODUCTION

Ginger is a common food item but has many health promoting activities. Some of these activities are attributed to small molecules. However, in many

---

* Corresponding author, Email: b021770@mailserv.cuhk.edu.hk, fax: 852 26035123, phone: 852 39436872.

cases the active principles have not been identified. In the following, the antioxidant activity of ginger is reviewed.

GINGER EXTRACTS, ESSENTIAL OIL, AND COMPOUNDS WITH ANTIOXIDANT ACTIVITY

Ghasemzadeh et al., (2010) compared the antioxidant activities of methanolic extracts of the leaves, rhizomes and stems of *Zingiber officinale* var. Halia Bentong and *Zingiber officinale* var. Halia Bara. The antioxidant activity and phenolic content of the leaves as measured by the 1,1-diphenyl-2-picryl-hydrazyl (DPPH) assay and the phenolic and flavonoid contents in the leaves were higher than those of the rhizomes and stems. The rhizome extract exhibited higher ferric reducing/antioxidant potential (FRAP) activity than the leaf extract. Halia Bara had higher antioxidant activity and phenolic and flavonoid contents than Halia Bentong. This investigation revealed the medicinal activity of the foliage and young rhizome of *Zingiber officinale* varieties and the correlation between total phenolics content and antioxidant activities in ginger (Ghasemzadeh et al., 2010).

Analysis of fresh and dried ginger volatile oils disclosed that camphene, p-cineole, alpha-terpineol, pentadecanoic acid and zingiberene are the principal constituents. High phenolic contents were found in the methanolic extract (95.2 mg/g dry extract) and the hexane extract (87.5 mg/g dry extract) of fresh ginger. Dried ginger and fresh ginger essential oils reduced ferric ions. Our data indicate that ginger is a potential source of natural antioxidants (El-Ghorab et al., 2010).

Alafiatayo et al. (2014) determined the total antioxidant capacity of ten species of Zingiberaceae (Ginger) which are employed as spices and medicine in Southeast Asia.

The results obtained revealed that methanol extracts of *Zingiber officinale* and *Curcuma longa* had the highest free radical scavenging capacity and ferric reducing power (Alafiatayo et al., 2014).

Alinkina et al. (2012) compared the antiradical properties of three samples of ginger including fresh rhizome juice, essential oil, and extracts (oleoresin) with the synthetic antioxidant ionol (butylatedhydroxy-toluene, BHT). The activities of ginger oleoresin and BHT were similar and same as those of highly active natural antioxidants. The activities of essential oil and ginger juice were lower by two orders of magnitude (Alinkina et al., 2012).

Twenty-nine phenolics isolated from the root bark of fresh Yunnan ginger were studied by Peng et al. (2012). Several diarylheptanoids and epoxidic diarylheptanoids were DPPH radical scavengers and xanthine oxidase inhibitors. An enone-dione analog of 6-shogaol potently protected PC12 cells from H_2O_2-induced damage. Almost all compounds were lipid peroxidation inhibitors. 6-shogaol, 10-gingerol and an enone-diarylheptanoid analog of curcumin were cytotoxic to the cell lines tested, with KB and HL60 cells being most susceptible to 6-shogaol and the curcumin analog with an IC_{50} below 10 μM (Peng et al., 2012).

ANTI-DIABETIC AND ANTI-OXIDANT EFFECTS

Aqueous extracts of raw ginger administered orally at 500 mg/ml for one month suppressed fasting blood glucose and malonydialdehyde levels, elevated serum insulin level and increased insulin sensitivity in alloxan-induced diabetic and insulin-resistant diabetic rats. One of the likely mechanisms is the action of malonydialdehyde, which acts as a scavenger of oxygen radical (Iranloye et al., 2011).

Feeding inbred male Wistar/NIN rats with ginger powder at 0.5%, 1% and 5% in diet for a month exerted a protective effect against streptozotocin - induced diabetes by modulating antioxidant enzymes and glutathione and downregulating lipid and protein oxidation and suppression of genotoxicity (Kota et al., 2012). The ethanolic ginger extract exerted low cytotoxicity toward INS-1E β cells and protective effects on viability of β cells, and downregulated oxidative stress markers (Račková et al., 2013).

Free and bound ginger polyphenols, especially the free polyphenols, could mitigate liver disorders caused by diabetes mellitus in rats as seen in changes in hepatic antioxidant enzymes, carbohydrate-metabolizing enzymes and liver function indices (Kazeem et al., 2013)

RELATIONSHIP BETWEEN TOTAL PHENOLIC CONTENT, ANTIOXIDANT POTENTIAL, AND ANTIGLYCATION ABILITIES

Ramkissoon et al., (2012) studied the total phenolic content, and antioxidant and antiglycation properties of crude ethanolic extracts of ten

Mauritius culinary herbs and spices. Ginger was found to have the most potent ferric-reducing antioxidant power. The antiglycation activities could not always be attributed to the phenolic content or antioxidant potential (Ramkissoon et al., 2012).

Beneficial Effects on Male Reproduction in Diabetic Rats

Sperm count, sperm viability, sperm motility, and serum testosterone level were elevated in diabetic rats treated with ginger, cinnamon, and a combination of ginger and cinnamon. Increased serum levels/activities of testosterone, FSH, LH, glutathione peroxidase, superoxide dismutase and catalase were observed. Combined treatment with ginger and cinnamon elicited more pronounced changes compared to treatment with ginger alone and cinnamon alone (Khaki et al., 2014).

Improvements in Semen Quality, Sperm Fatty Acids, and Reproductive Performance in Old Roosters

Ginger powder, rich in antioxidative compounds, was fed to 52-wk-old Cobb 500 breeder roosters for 14 weeks at 15 or 30 g /kg diet. The treatment improved sperm forward motility, sperm viability, and sperm plasma membrane integrity. The concentration of thiobarbituric acid reactive species and percentage of abnormal sperms in the semen were reduced while the total antioxidant capacity in seminal plasma and the number of perivitelline membrane sperm penetration holes were increased although there were no changes in hatchability, chick quality, and embryonic mortality (Akhlaghi et al., 2014).

Antidepressant-Like Activity

Dehydrozingerone is a phenolic compound isolated from ginger rhizomes known for its antioxidant, anti-inflammatory and antitumor activities. Its potent antidepressant effect involves the serotonergic and noradrenergic systems (Martinez et al., 2014).

Anti-Alzheimer Effects

The methanolic extract of dry ginger expressed high antioxidant activity and cholinesterase inhibitory activity It increased survival of adult rat hippocampal cells in primary culture against amyloid beta (Abeta) induced toxicity. The methanolic extract prevented the formation of Abeta oligomers and dissociated the preformed oligomers. Thus the methanolic extract can be used as a neutraceutical supplement for Alzheimer's disease (Mathew and Subramanian, 2014).

Protective Effect against Oxidative Stress in the Brain

Neurodegenerative diseases are believed to be associated with oxidative stress caused by peroxidation of membrane biomolecules and a high Fe level. Incubation of rat brain tissue homogenate in the presence of Fe resulted in an increase of lipid peroxidation as evidenced by a rise in the end-product, malondialdehyde. The aqueous extract of red ginger (*Zingiber officinale* var. Rubra) suppressed Fe(2+)-induced lipid peroxidation in the rat brain with a higher efficacy than the aqueous extract of white ginger (*Zingiber officinale* Roscoe) probably because of a higher phytochemical content, reducing power, hydroxyl radical scavenging activity, and Fe(2+) chelating activity. Thus, consumption of ginger may help reduce oxidative stress in the brain (Oboh et al., 2010).

Gastroprotective Activity

'Kissing' ulcers were induced in male Sprague-Dawley rats with 60% acetic acid. Oral administration of ginger extract (1.5-5 g/kg/day) and polaprezinc (30 and 60 mg/kg/day) for 3 days following ulcer induction brought about a decrease in the ulcerated area, activities of xanthine oxidase and myeloperoxidase, and malondialdehyde level in the ulcerated mucosa.

Only the mucosal glutathione level was only restored by polaprezinc. Both polaprezinc and ginger extract upregulated the expression of vascular endothelial growth factor and basic fibroblast growth factor, while ornithine decarboxylase was increased only by polaprezinc in the gastric mucosa. Polaprezinc downregulated protein expression of cytokine-induced neutrophil chemoattractant-2á, tumor necrosis factor-á, macrophage inflammatory protein-2, and interleukin-1âin the ulcerated tissues, whereas ginger extract suppressed the expression of the chemokines and to some extent tumor necrosis factor-á. Hence both ginger extract and polaprezinc manifest anti-oxidative activity which mitigates gastric mucosal damage and enhances ulcer healing (Ko and Leung, 2010).

Ginger essential oil could reduce ethanol- induced gastric ulcer in rat stomach as seen from the ulcer index and gastric histopathology and restored the activities of antioxidant enzymes such as glutathione peroxidase, superoxide dismutase, catalase and glutathione levels (Liju et al., 2014).

Protection against Nephrotoxicity Induced by CCl4

Hamed et al., (2012) assessed successive ginger extracts (petroleum ether, chloroform, and ethanol) for protection against nephrotoxicity induced by CCl4 in rats. Treatment with ginger extracts, especially the ethanol extract, drastically reduced levels of lipid peroxides, prostaglandin-E2, collagen and kidney function (urea, creatinine) tests, and upregulated levels of glutathione, superoxide dismutase and serum protein (Hamed et al., 2012).

Antioxidant Activity on Various Organs

Misharina et al., (2014) investigated the actions of oregano and clove essential oils and a mixture of lemon essential oil and a ginger extract on the antioxidant status of murine organs. All essential oils suppressed lipid peroxidation in erythrocyte membranes leading to enhanced membrane resistance to spontaneous hemolysis, reduced membrane microviscosity, maintenance of their structural integrity, and functional activity. The essential oils reduced lipid peroxidation in the liver and the brains and increased resistance of their lipids to oxidation and upregulated the activities of hepatic antioxidant enzymes (Misharina et al., 2014).

INHIBITION OF HUMAN LOW-DENSITY LIPOPROTEIN OXIDATION

Oxidative modification of low-density lipoprotein (LDL) plays a paramount role in atherosclerotic plaque formation. Ethanol, methanol, ethyl acetate, hexane and water extracts of ginger inhibited LDL oxidation by 71%, 76%, 67%, 67% and 43%, respectively. Phenolic bioactives of ginger-6-gingerols, 8-gingerols, 10-gingerols, and 6-shogaol potently inhibited Cu(+2)-induced LDL oxidation (Gunathilake and Rupasinghe, 2014).

EFFECT ON SKIN CELL GROWTH

10-shogaol from ginger exhibited antioxidant activity in the 1,1-diphenyl-2-picrylhydrazyl (DPPH) radical scavenging assay, metal chelating assay,, and reducing power assay.. 10-Shogaol exerted a growth promoting action on human normal epidermal keratinocytes and dermal fibroblasts. 10-Shogaol stimulated production of transforming growth factor-â, platelet derived growth factor-áâ, and vascular endothelial growth factors in both types of cells, and the migration of fibroblasts and keratinocytes in the *in vitro* wound healing assay. Thus, 10-shogaol serves as an antioxidant for human skin cell growth and a migration enhancer and a potential wound repair agent (Chen et al., 2012).

AMELIORATION OF PESTICIDE TOXICITY

Lindane administration (30 mg/kg bw orally for 4 weeks) to rats increased lipid peroxidation and attenuated antioxidant defense. Dietary inclusion of ginger (1%w/w) inhibited lindane-induced lipid peroxidation, escorted by modulation of superoxide dismutase and catalase as well as reduced glutathione and glutathione peroxidase, glutathione reductase and glutathione-S-transferase (Ahmed et al., 2008).

Administration of dichlorvos alone, lindane alone, and dichlorvos in conjunction with lindane, increased lipid peroxidation and decreased the reduced glutathione level, superoxide dismutase, catalase, glutathione peroxidase, glutathione S-transferase, glutathione reductase, quinine reductase and protein in the rat brain. Oxidative stress due to abnormal production of reactive oxygen species is implicated in the toxic action of the two pesticides. Ginger juice treatment ameliorated the changes (Sharma and Singh, 2012).

Antioxidant Activity in Broilers

All broiler chicks receiving dietary ginger powder and essential oil had increased total antioxidant capacity and decreased malondialdehyde concentration in serum compared to the control group. Ginger powder and essential oil may be a suitable replacement for synthetic antioxidants in broiler diets and ginger powder might be better than essential oil for improving antioxidant status in broilers (Habibi et al., 2014).

Conclusion

The foregoing account reveals that many of the actions of ginger such as antidiabetic, neuroprotective, gastroprotective, nephroprotective, gastroprotective, and cardioprotective actions of ginger are related to its antioxidant activity. In fact, it has been hypothesized that aging, neurodegeneration, cardiovascular diseases, and cancer etc. are associated with oxidative stress. Antioxidants such as vitamin C, vitamin E, and melatonin are beneficial to health. Compared with other food items, ginger is relatively cheap. Dietary consumption of ginger is recommended.

References

Abdel-Azeem AS, Hegazy AM, Ibrahim KS, Farrag AR, El-Sayed EM. Hepatoprotective, antioxidant, and ameliorative effects of ginger (Zingiber officinale Roscoe) and vitamin E in acetaminophen treated rats. *J Diet Suppl.* 2013;10(3):195-209.

Ademiluyi AO, Oboh G, Ogunsuyi OB, Akinyemi AJ. Attenuation of gentamycin-induced nephrotoxicity in rats by dietary inclusion of ginger (Zingiber officinale) and turmeric (Curcuma longa) rhizomes. *Nutr Health.* 2012;21(4):209-18.

Ahmed RS, Suke SG, Seth V, Chakraborti A, Tripathi AK, Banerjee BD. Protective effects of dietary ginger (Zingiber officinales Rosc.) on lindane-induced oxidative stress in rats. *Phytother Res.* 2008;22(7):902-6.

Akhlaghi A, Ahangari YJ, Navidshad B, Pirsaraei ZA, Zhandi M, Deldar H, Rezvani MR, Dadpasand M, Hashemi SR, Poureslami R, Peebles ED. Improvements in semen quality, sperm fatty acids, and reproductive performance in aged Cobb 500 breeder roosters fed diets containing dried ginger rhizomes (Zingiber officinale). *Poult Sci.* 2014;93(5):1236-44.

Alafiatayo AA, Syahida A, Mahmood M. Total anti-oxidant capacity, flavonoid, phenolic acid and polyphenol content in ten selected species of Zingiberaceae rhizomes. *Afr J Tradit Complement Altern Med.* 2014;11(3):7-13.

Alinkina ES, Misharina TA, Fatkullina LD, Burlakova EB. Comparison of the antiradical activity of ionol, components of fresh ginger, and its extracts. *Prikl Biokhim Mikrobiol.* 2012;48(5):564-9.

Bak MJ, Ok S, Jun M, Jeong WS. 6-shogaol-rich extract from ginger up-regulates the antioxidant defense systems in cells and mice. *Molecules.* 2012 Jul 4;17(7):8037-55.

Chen CY, Cheng KC, Chang AY, Lin YT, Hseu YC, Wang HM. 10-Shogaol, an antioxidant from Zingiber officinale for skin cell proliferation and migration enhancer. *Int J Mol Sci.* 2012;13(2):1762-77.

El-Ghorab AH, Nauman M, Anjum FM, Hussain S, Nadeem M. A comparative study on chemical composition and antioxidant activity of ginger (Zingiber officinale) and cumin (Cuminum cyminum). *J Agric Food Chem.* 2010;58(14):8231-7.

Ghasemzadeh A, Jaafar HZ, Rahmat A. Antioxidant activities, total phenolics and flavonoids content in two varieties of Malaysia young ginger (Zingiber officinale Roscoe). *Molecules.* 2010;15(6):4324-33.

Ghlissi Z, Atheymen R, Boujbiha MA, Sahnoun Z, Makni Ayedi F, Zeghal K, El Feki A, Hakim A. Antioxidant and androgenic effects of dietary ginger on reproductive function of male diabetic rats. *Int J Food Sci Nutr.* 2013;64(8):974-8.

Gunathilake KD, Rupasinghe HP. Inhibition of human low-density lipoprotein oxidation in vitro by ginger extracts. *J Med Food.* 2014;17(4):424-31.

Habibi R, Sadeghi G, Karimi A. Effect of different concentrations of ginger root powder and its essential oil on growth performance, serum metabolites and antioxidant status in broiler chicks under heat stress. *Br Poult Sci.* 2014;55(2):228-37.

Hamed MA, Ali SA, El-Rigal NS. Therapeutic potential of ginger against renal injury induced by carbon tetrachloride in rats. *Scientific World Journal.* 2012;2012:840421.

Iranloye BO, Arikawe AP, Rotimi G, Sogbade AO. Anti-diabetic and anti-oxidant effects of Zingiber officinale on alloxan-induced and insulin-resistant diabetic male rats. *Niger J Physiol Sci.* 2011;26(1):89-96.

Jeena K, Liju VB, Kuttan R.Antioxidant, anti-inflammatory and antinociceptive activities of essential oil from ginger. *Indian J Physiol Pharmacol.* 2013;57(1):51-62.

Jittiwat J, Wattanathorn J. Ginger pharmacopuncture improves cognitive impairment and oxidative stress following cerebral ischemia. *J Acupunct Meridian Stud.* 2012;5(6):295-300.

Kazeem MIAkanji MAYakubu MT, Ashafa AO Protective Effect of Free and Bound Polyphenol Extracts from Ginger (Zingiber officinale Roscoe) on the Hepatic Antioxidant and Some Carbohydrate Metabolizing Enzymes of Streptozotocin-Induced Diabetic Rats. *Evid Based Complement Alternat Med.* 2013;2013:935486.

Khaki A, Khaki AA, Hajhosseini L, Golzar FS, Ainehchi N. The Anti-Oxidant Effects of Ginger and Cinnamon on Spermatogenesis Dys-function of Diabetes Rats. *Afr J Tradit Complement Altern Med.* 2014;11(4):1-8.

Ko JK, Leung CC. Ginger extract and polaprezinc exert gastroprotective actions by anti-oxidant and growth factor modulating effects in rats. *J Gastroenterol Hepatol.* 2010;25(12):1861-8.

Kota N, Panpatil VV, Kaleb R, Varanasi B, Polasa K. Dose-dependent effect in the inhibition of oxidative stress and anticlastogenic potential of ginger in STZ induced diabetic rats. *Food Chem.* 2012;135(4):2954-9.

Kubra IR, Bettadaiah BK, Murthy PS, Rao LJ. Structure-function activity of dehydrozingerone and its derivatives as antioxidant and antimicrobial compounds. *J Food Sci Technol.* 2014;51(2):245-55.

Li F, Nitteranon V, Tang X, Liang J, Zhang G, Parkin KL, Hu Q. In vitro antioxidant and anti-inflammatory activities of 1-dehydro-[6]-gingerdione, 6-shogaol, 6-dehydroshogaol and hexahydrocurcumin. *Food Chem.* 2012;135(2):332-7.

Liju VB, Jeena K, Kuttan R. Gastroprotective activity of essential oils from turmeric and ginger. *J Basic Clin Physiol Pharmacol.* 2014 Apr 21. [Epub ahead of print]

Manjunatha JR, Bettadaiah BK, Negi PS, Srinivas P. Synthesis of quinoline derivatives of tetrahydrocurcumin and zingerone and evaluation of their antioxidant and antibacterial attributes. *Food Chem.* 2013;136(2):650-8.

Martinez DM, Barcellos A, Casaril AM, Savegnago L, Lernardão EJ. Antidepressant-like activity of dehydrozingerone: Involvement of the serotonergic and noradrenergic systems. *Pharmacol Biochem Behav.* 2014;127C:111-117.

Mashhadi NS, Ghiasvand R, Hariri M, Askari G, Feizi A, Darvishi L, Hajishafiee M, Barani A. Effect of ginger and cinnamon intake on oxidative stress and exercise performance and body composition in Iranian female athletes. *Int J Prev Med.* 2013;4(Suppl 1):S31-5.

Mathew M, Subramanian S. In vitro evaluation of anti-Alzheimer effects of dry ginger (Zingiber officinale Roscoe) extract. *Indian J Exp Biol.* 2014;52(6):606-12.

Misharina TA, Fatkullina LD, Alinkina ES, Kozachenko AI, Nagler LG, Medvedeva IB, Goloshchapov AN, Burlakova EB. Effects of low doses of essential oil on the antioxidant state of the erythrocytes, liver, and the brains of mice. *Prikl Biokhim Mikrobiol.* 2014;50(1):101-7.

Oboh G, Akinyemi AJ, Ademiluyi AO. Antioxidant and inhibitory effect of red ginger (Zingiber officinale var. Rubra) and white ginger (Zingiber officinale Roscoe) on Fe(2+) induced lipid peroxidation in rat brain in vitro. *Exp Toxicol Pathol.* 2012;64(1-2):31-6.

Peng F, Tao Q, Wu X, Dou H, Spencer S, Mang C, Xu L, Sun L, Zhao Y, Li H, Zeng S, Liu G, Hao X. Cytotoxic, cytoprotective and antioxidant effects of isolated phenolic compounds from fresh ginger. *Fitoterapia.* 2012;83(3):568-85.

Račková L, Cupáková M, Tažký A, Mičová J, Kolek E, Košťálová D. Redox properties of ginger extracts: Perspectives of use of Zingiber officinale Rosc. as antidiabetic agent. *Interdiscip Toxicol.* 2013;6(1):26-33.

Ramkissoon JS, Mahomoodally MF, Ahmed N, Subratty AH. Relationship between total phenolic content, antioxidant potential, and antiglycation abilities of common culinary herbs and spices. *J Med Food.* 2012;15(12):1116-23.

Shanmugam KR, Ramakrishna CH, Mallikarjuna K, Reddy KS. Protective effect of ginger against alcohol-induced renal damage and antioxidant enzymes in male albino rats. *Indian J Exp Biol.* 2010;48(2):143-9.

Sharma P, Singh R. Dichlorvos and lindane induced oxidative stress in rat brain: Protective effects of ginger. *Pharmacognosy Res.* 2012;4(1):27-32.

In: Ginger
Editor: Janine L. Perry
ISBN: 978-1-63482-020-2

Chapter 4

MEDICINAL EFFECTS OF GINGER

Tzi Bun Ng* and Charlene Cheuk Wing Ng
School of Biomedical Sciences, Faculty of Medicine,
The Chinese University of Hong Kong, New Territories, Hong Kong,China

ABSTRACT

Ginger displays protective effects on Alzheimer's disease. It brings about attenuation of neuroinflammation and cognitive deficits. It exhibits anti-inflammatory, anticancer, antihypercholesterolemic, hepato-protective, anti-rheumatoid arthritis, antinociceptive, anti-viral, anti-schistosomal and insecticidal activities. It inhibits bacterial biofilm formation. It prevents nausea and vomiting, and exerts a protective effect on the metabolic syndrome-associated kidney injury. It decreases the severity of symptoms of premenstrual syndrome.

INTRODUCTION

Ginger is the rhizome of the plant *Zingiber officinale*. It is used for cooking and also in traditional medicine. Its various biological activities account for its use in traditional medicine in various countries. The chemical

* Corresponding author, Email: b021770@mailserv.cuhk.edu.hk, fax: 852 26035123, phone: 852 39436872.

identity of only some of the principles responsible for the biological activities has been elucidated.

ALZHEIMER'S DISEASE

Azam et al., (2014) undertook molecular docking investigations to study the binding interactions between active ginger components and various anti-Alzheimer drug targets. Lamarckian genetic algorithm methodology was used for docking of twelve ligands with thirteen target proteins using AutoDock 4.2 program. Validation of docking protocol was performed by re-docking of all native co-crystallized ligands into their original binding cavities showing a high correlation coefficient (r (2)=0.931) between docking predicted and experimentally activities. The value of the coefficient indicates that the methodology could be employed as a computational tool to facilitate optimization of ginger lead compounds. Analysis of binding energy, predicted inhibition constant and hydrophobic/hydrophilic interactions of ligands with target receptors demonstrated that acetylcholinesterase was the most promising, whereas c-Jun N-terminal kinase was as the least favorable anti-Alzheimer's drug target. Common structural requirements comprise hydrogen bond donor/acceptor area, hydrophobic domain, carbon spacer, and distal hydrophobic domain flanked by hydrogen bond donor/acceptor moieties. Drug-likeness score and molecular properties desired of a good pharmacokinetic profile were computed by Osiris property explorer and Molinspiration online toolkit, respectively. None of the compounds violated Lipinski's rule of five. Thus they are potentially good therapeutic candidates for Alzheimer's disease (Azam et al., 2014).

PROTECTIVE EFFECTS ON ALZHEIMER DISEASE-INDUCED BEHAVIORAL DYSFUNCTION

Zeng et al., (2013) established a rat model of Alzheimer disease by using an operation in which amyloid β-protein was injected intracerebroventricularly into the rats which were then treated with a continuous gavage of aluminum chloride daily for a month. Ginger root extract was administered intragastrically. Thirty-five days later, learning and memory in the animals were evaluated. Brain sections were processed for immunohistochemistry and staining. The latency to show significant memory deficits was shorter, the expression levels of catalase and superoxide dismutase were weaker, and the expression levels of nuclear factor-κB, interleukin-1β, and malondialdehyde were lower, in the group that received a high dose of ginger root extract than in the groups that received a low or moderate dose of ginger root extract. This experiment demonstrates that treatment with ginger root extract reverses behavioral dysfunction and prevents Alzheimer disease-like symptoms in rats (Zeng et al., 2013).

Attenuation of Neuroinflammation and Cognitive Deficits

6-Shogaol exerted anti-neuroinflammatory effects in lipopolysaccharide - treated astrocytes and animal models of Parkinson's disease, lipopolysaccharide-induced inflammation and transient global ischemia. It decreased microgliosis and astrogliosis in intrahippocampal AβO-injected mice, ameliorated AβO and scopolamine-induced memory impairment, and raised levels of nerve growth factor and hippocampal pre-and post-synaptic marker. 6-shogaol may suppress glial cell activation and mitigate memory impairment in animal dementia models (Moon et al., 2014).

Antiinflammatory Activity

Traditionally, ginger is used as an anti-inflammatory drug. The effects of a ginger extract and some ginger compounds on lipopolysaccharide -induced secretion of interleukin 8 and RANTES (regulated upon activation, normal T-cell expressed and secreted) in human bronchial epithelial cells (BEAS-2B cells) were tested. An oily extract of ginger rhizome with over 25% total pungent compounds, and ginger volatile oil, undermined the lipopolysaccharide–induced release of the proinflammatory chemokine interleukin 8. The pungent [6]-gingerol and its metabolite [6]-shogaol were inactive. The ginger volatile oil inhibited lipopolysaccharide-timulated rise of RANTES. Hence some ginger compounds could be utilized to treat inflammation in respiratory infections (Podlogar and Verspohl, 2012).

Anticancer Activity

[6]-gingerol, the major active principle of ginger, was non-toxic toward normal mouse colon cells but suppressed cell proliferation and induced apoptosis in SW-480 human colon cancer cells. Sensitivity to [6]-gingerol in SW-480 cells was associated with activation of caspases 8, 9, 3 and 7 and PARP cleavage. [6]-gingerol reduced phorbol myristate acetate-induced ERK1/2 and JNK MAP kinase phosphorylation and AP-1 transcription factor activation, but was devoid of action on NF-kappa B activation and p38 MAP kinase phosphorylation. [6]-gingerol complemented the inhibitors of either ERK1/2 or JNK MAP kinase in suppressing phorbol myristate acetate-induced cell proliferation in SW-480 cells. Hence the suppression of ERK1/2/JNK/AP-1 pathway is a likely mechanism underlying the antitumor and chemopreventive actions of [6]-gingerol against colon cancer (Radhakrishnan et al., 2014).

The cancer chemopreventive effects of [6]-gingerol, and its inhibitory effect on various stages of the process of metastasis have been reviewed by Poltronieri et al. (2014).

Antihypercholesterolaemic Effect

Hypercholesterolaemic rats treated with an aqueous ginger infusion for 2 and 4 weeks manifested reduced levels of serum total cholesterol, low density lipoprotein cholesterol, and triglyceride (ElRokh et al., 2010).

Hepatoprotective Effect

An ethanolic extract of ginger rhizomes protected against thioacetamide-induced hepatotoxicity in rats and reduced hepatic fibrosis. Immunohistochemical assessment against proliferating cell nuclear antigen failed to reveal significant proliferation in the ginger-treated rats. Fractions derived from the ginger extract manifested antiproliferative activity toward hepatoma Hep-G2 cells (Abdulaziz Bardi et al., 2013).

Oral administration of free and bound ginger polyphenols to streptozotocin-induced diabetic rats brought about a decline in the fasting blood glucose level, and a rise in the activities of antioxidant enzymes, normalization of the activities of hepatic hexokinase and phosphofructokinase, and a decline in the activities of hepatic aminotransferases enzymes. Thus ginger ameliorated hepatic problems induced by diabetes mellitus (Kazeem et al., 2013).

Protective Effect on the Metabolic Syndrome-Associated Kidney Injury

Ginger supplementation in rats with ethanolic extract of ginger (50 mg/kg) improved hyperinsulinemia and hypertriglyceridemia, reduced fructose (10% fructose in drinking water over 5 weeks)-induced renal damage through suppression of fructose-stimulated monocyte chemoattractant protein-1 and its receptor chemokine (C-C motif) receptor-2, overexpression of two important macrophage accumulation markers CD68 and F4/80 and overexpression of macrophage-associated proinflammatory cytokines tumor necrosis factor-alpha, interleukin-6, transforming growth factor-beta1 and plasminogen activator inhibitor in rats. Renal damage characterized by focal cast formation, slough and dilation of tubular epithelial cells in the renal cortex and excessive renal interstitial collagen deposit was reduced. The results signify that ginger protects against kidney injury associated with the metabolic syndrome (Yang et al., 2014).

Anti-Rheumatoid Arthritis Effect

A mixture of ginger and turmeric rhizomes powder (1:1) suspended in distilled water displayed higher efficacy than the nonsteroidal anti-inflammatory drug indomethacin in mitigating the loss in body weight gain, histopathological alterations in ankle joints, blood leukocytosis and thrombocytosis, iron deficiency anemia, serum hypoalbuminemia and globulinemia, renal impairment, and cardiovascular disease risks in arthritic rats. These protective effects of the ginger and turmeric mixture were mediated through elevating food consumption and decreasing the systemic inflammation at the appearance of polyarthritis, oxidative stress and dyslipidemia (Ramadan and El-Menshawy, 2013).

Prevention of Nausea and Vomiting

Ginger has been employed as an antiemetic in traditional medicine for centuries. Its antiemetic effects against various emetogenic stimuli have been demonstrated in preclinical and clinical studies. However, results on the prevention of chemotherapy induced nausea and vomiting and motion sickness were not in concord (Palatty et al., 2013).

Antinociceptive Effect

The essential oil of Zingiber zerumbet, a wild edible ginger species, when administered intraperitoneally and orally at 50, 100, 200 and 300 mg/kg, demonstrated antinociceptive activity in chemical-induced murine nociception tests including acetic acid-induced abdominal constriction test, and paw licking test induced by capsaicin-,glutamate- and phorbol 12-myristate 13-acetate Involvement of the l-arginine/nitric oxide pathway was suggested by the reversal of antinociception by pretreatment with l-arginine, a precursor of nitric oxide. Reversal of antinociception induced by ginger essential oil was also effected by treatment with glibenclamide, an ATP-sensitive K(+) channel antagonist. Augmentation of antinociception was brought about by methylene blue. The antinociceptive activity was probably related to suppression of the glutamatergic system, TRPV1 receptors and mediated by activation of l-arginine/nitric oxide/cGMP/protein kinase C/ATP-sensitive K(+) channel pathway (Khalid et al., 2011).

Decreasing the Severity of Symptoms of Premenstrual Syndrome

Khayat et al. (2014) conducted a double-blind clinical trial in which there were 35 subjects in each of the control group and the intervention group. To identify premenstrual syndrome, the subjects had to fill out a daily record scale questionnaire for two consecutive cycles. The subjects so identified received two ginger capsules daily for three cycles, starting one week prior to menstruation to three days post-menstruation. Severity of the symptoms was noted down by a daily record scale questionnaire. Pre-intervention results were compared with data 1, 2, and 3 months post-intervention. Ginger is probably effective in decreasing the severity of mood and physical and behavioral symptoms of premenstrual syndrome (Khayat et al., 2014).

Inhibition of Bacterial Biofilm Formation

Bacterial biofilm formation can cause serious problems clinically and industrially.

A static Pseudomonas aeruginosa PA14 biofilm assay demonstrated that biofilm development decreased by 39-56% after addition of ginger extract. Ginger extract suppressed formation of extracellular polymeric substances. In the presence of ginger extract, less rugose colonies were formed on agar plates containing Congo red and swarming motility on soft agar plates was facilitated. The suppression of biofilm formation and the altered phenotypes were related to a diminished concentration of a second messenger, bis-(3'-5')-cyclic dimeric guanosine monophosphate. Ginger extract suppressed biofilm formation in both Gram-positive and Gram-negative bacteria. Also, surface biofilm cells formed in the presence of ginger extract were more easily detached with surfactant than those formed in the absence of ginger extract (Kim and Park, 2013).

Anti-Viral Activity

Hot water extract of fresh but not dried ginger dose-dependently suppressed human respiratory syncytial virus-induced plaque formation in both human upper (HEp-2) and low (A549) respiratory tract cell lines. A higher efficacy was observed when it was administered prior to viral inoculation. Fresh ginger also prevented viral attachment and internalization, and upregulated interferon-β production by mucosal cells (Chang et al., 2013).

Antischistosomal Activity

C57 mice with or without ginger treatment and exposed to 100 ± 10 Schistosoma mansoni cercariae per mouse by the tail immersion method were sacrificed 10 weeks after infection. The ginger-treated mice exhibited a lower worm burden and egg density in liver and feces than in untreated mice. Male worms recovered from ginger-treated mice displayed partial loss of tubercles' spines, massive erosion in inter-tubercle tegumental regions and many tiny blebs surrounding the tubercles. The number and size of hepatic and intestinal granulomatous inflammatory infiltrations in treated mice were reduced compared with untreated mice (Mostafa et al., 2011).

INSECTICIDAL ACTIVITY

Ginger essential oil reduced oviposition and hatching rate and caused contact toxicity in adults of the beetle *Callosobruchus chinensis* and it could be used in insect pest management (Chaubey, 2013).

DISCUSSION

The foregoing account reveals that ginger manifests a diversity of exploitable activities. The principles eliciting some of the aforementioned activities, e.g. insecticidal, antischistosomal, anti-viral activity and inhibition of bacterial biofilm formation decreased the severity of symptoms of premenstrual syndrome, antinociceptive effect, prevented nausea and vomiting; hepatoprotective effect and antihypercholesterolemic effect remain to be isolated and chemically characterized. This may disclose novel compounds.

REFERENCES

Abdulaziz Bardi D, Halabi MF, Abdullah NA, Rouhollahi E, Hajrezaie M, Abdulla MA. In vivo evaluation of ethanolic extract of Zingiber officinale rhizomes for its protective effect against liver cirrhosis. *Biomed Res Int.* 2013;2013:918460.

Azam F, Amer AM, Abulifa AR, Elzwawi MM. Ginger components as new leads for the design and development of novelmulti-targeted anti-Alzheimer's drugs: a computational investigation. *Drug Des Devel Ther.* 2014;8:2045-59.

Chang JS, Wang KC, Yeh CF, Shieh DE, Chiang LC. Fresh ginger (Zingiber officinale) has anti-viral activity against human respiratory syncytial virus in human respiratory tract cell lines. *J Ethnopharmacol.* 2013;145(1):146-51.

Chaubey MK Biological activities of Zingiber officinale (Zingiberaceae) and Piper cubeba (Piperaceae) essential oils against pulse beetle, Callosobruchus chinensis (Coleoptera: Bruchidae). *Pak J Biol Sci.* 2013;16(11):517-23.

ElRokh el-SM, Yassin NA, El-Shenawy SM, Ibrahim BM. Antihypercholesterolaemic effect of ginger rhizome (Zingiber officinale) in rats. *Inflammopharmacology.* 2010;18(6):309-15.

Kazeem MI, Akanji MA, Yakubu MT, Ashafa AO. Protective Effect of Free and Bound Polyphenol Extracts from Ginger (Zingiber officinale Roscoe) on the Hepatic Antioxidant and Some Carbohydrate Metabolizing Enzymes of Streptozotocin Induced Diabetic Rats. *Evid Based Complement Alternat Med.* 2013;2013:935486.

Khalid MH, Akhtar MN, Mohamad AS, Perimal EK, Akira A, Israf DA, Lajis N, Sulaiman MR. Antinociceptive effect of the essential oil of Zingiber zerumbet in mice:possible mechanisms. *J Ethnopharmacol.* 2011;137(1):345-51.

Khayat S Kheirkhah M, Behboodi Moghadam Z, Fanaei H, Kasaeian A, Javadimehr M.Effect of treatment with ginger on the severity of premenstrual syndrome symptoms. I*SRN Obstet Gynecol.* 2014;2014:792708.

Kim HS, Park HD. Ginger extract inhibits biofilm formation by Pseudomonas aeruginosa PA14. *PLoS One.* 2013;8(9):e76106.

Moon M, Kim HG, Choi JG, Oh H, Lee PK, Ha SK, Kim SY, Park Y, Huh Y, Oh MS. 6-Shogaol, an active constituent of ginger, attenuates neuroinflammation and cognitive deficits in animal models of dementia. *Biochem Biophys Res Commun.* 2014;449(1):8-13.

Mostafa OM, Eid RA, Adly MA. Antischistosomal activity of ginger (Zingiber officinale) against Schistosoma mansoni harbored in C57 mice. *Parasitol Res.* 2011;109(2):395-403.

Palatty PL, Haniadka R, Valder B, Arora R, Baliga MS. Ginger in the prevention of nausea and vomiting: a review. *Crit Rev Food Sci Nutr.* 2013;53(7):659-69.

Podlogar JA, Verspohl EJ. Antiinflammatory effects of ginger and some of its components in human bronchial epithelial (BEAS-2B) cells. *Phytother Res.* 2012;26(3):333-6.

Poltronieri J, Becceneri AB, Fuzer AM, Filho JC, Martin AC, Vieira PC, Pouliot N, Cominetti MR. [6]-gingerol as a cancer chemopreventive agent: a review of its activity on different steps of the metastatic process. *Mini Rev Med Chem*. 2014;14(4):313-21.

Radhakrishnan EK, Bava SV, Narayanan SS, Nath LR, Thulasidasan AK, Soniya EV, Anto RJ. [6]-Gingerol induces caspase-dependent apoptosis and prevents PMA-induced proliferation in colon cancer cells by inhibiting MAPK/AP-1 signaling. *PLoS One*. 2014 Aug 26;9(8):e104401.

Rahmani AH, Shabrmi FM, Aly SM. Active ingredients of ginger as potential candidates in the prevention and treatment of diseases via modulation of biological activities. *Int J Physiol Pathophysiol Pharmacol*. 2014;6(2):125-36.

Ramadan G, El-Menshawy O. Protective effects of ginger-turmeric rhizomes mixture on joint inflammation,atherogenesis, kidney dysfunction and other complications in a rat model of human rheumatoid arthritis. *Int J Rheum Dis*. 2013;16(2):219-29.

Yang M, Liu C, Jiang J, Zuo G, Lin X, Yamahara J, Wang J, Li Y. Ginger extract diminishes chronic fructose consumption-induced kidney injury through suppression of renal overexpression of proinflammatory cytokines in rats. *BMC Complement Altern Med*. 2014;14:174.

Zeng GF, Zhang ZY, Lu L, Xiao DQ, Zong SH, He JM. Protective effects of ginger root extract on Alzheimer disease-induced behavioral dysfunction in rats. *Rejuvenation Res*. 2013;16(2):124-33.

In: Ginger
Editor: Janine L. Perry

ISBN: 978-1-63482-020-2

Chapter 5

6-GINGEROL: BIOSYNTHESIS, CHEMISTRY AND POTENTIAL CARDIOVASCULAR HEALTH BENEFITS OF A GINGER BIOACTIVE

K. D. P. P. Gunathilake[1]
and H. P. Vasantha Rupasinghe[2]
[1]Department of Food Science & Technology,
Faculty of Livestock, Fisheries & Nutrition
Wayamba University of Sri Lanka, Makandura, Gonawila, Sri Lanka
[2]Department of Environmental Sciences,
Faculty of Agriculture, Dalhousie University, Truro, Canada

ABSTRACT

Ginger is a world known food plant which is equally reputed for its food flavoring and medicinal properties. 6-Gingerol is the major phenolic plant secondary metabolite present in the rhizome of ginger. This chapter reports chemical structure, biosynthesis, analytical methods and pharmacology as well as most recent research findings on potential cardiovascular health benefits of 6-gingerol. Qualitative and quantitative analytical techniques for the analysis of 6-gingerol and for the determination of the metabolism and bioavailability of 6-gingerol are discussed. Analytical techniques used for 6-gingerol that are described in this chapter are thin-layer chromatography (TLC), high-performance liquid chromatography (HPLC) combined with various detectors, and nuclear magnetic resonance (NMR) spectroscopy. The potential cardiovascular health effects of 6-gingerol include, anti-atherosclerotic, anti-platelet aggregation and antihypertensive effects as well as fibrinolytic activity.

1. INTRODUCTION

Ginger (*Zingiber officinale* Roscoe) has been used not only as a seasoning spice but also as an important phyto-medicine all around the world especially in Asia and Africa. The major bioactive constituents in ginger are the so called ''pungent principles'', the gingerols (Figure 1) of which 6-gingerol is the most abundant (Gupta & Sharma, 2014; Wang et al., 2011; Ali et al., 2008). Gingerols thought to be the most pharmacologically active component in ginger (Kim et al., 2005). [6]-Gingeol displays diverse biological activities such as anticancer (Bode et al., 2001; Katiyar, et al., 1996; Shukla & Singh, 2007), anti-oxidation (Masuda et al., 2004), anti-inflammation (Lam et al., 2007; Minghetti et al., 2007), inhibition of cyclooxygenase -2 (COX-2) expression (Li et al, 2013; Kim et al., 2004, 2005, 2007), antifungal (Ficker et al.,2003), anti-platelet aggregation (Hibino et al., 2008; Nie et al., 2008) activities among many others. Numerous research have been carried out on ginger during the last decades in order to develop analytical method for the identification, quantification of gingerols, as well as for the determination of metabolism and pharmacokinetics in humans. For the analysis of ginger bioactives including 6-gingerol, various chromatographic methods have been used. The bioactivity of [6]-gingerol has been widely investigated in relation to its medicinal properties. There have been various attempts to understand the mechanisms by which [6]-gingerol affect lipid and energy metabolism (Singh et al., 2009).

Some studies using cell culture systems have been shown that [6]-gingerol to be the active principle of ginger (Ali et al., 2008). Gingerols have high industrial applications in the development of food ingredients, additives, natural health products and even medicine. The aim of this chapter is to review the current status of the knowledge on chemistry, biosynthesis, analytical methods and the potential cardiovascular health effects of [6]-gingerol.

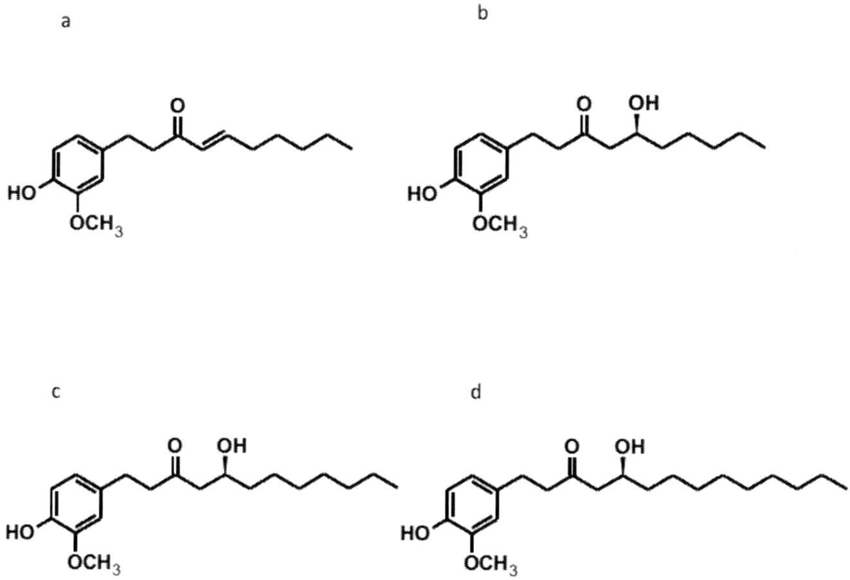

Figure 1. Structures of selected major bioactives of ginger: 6-shogaol (a), 6-gingerol (b), 8-gingerol (c), 10-gingerol (d) present in ginger.

2. CHEMISTRY

A. Chemical Structure of [6]-Gingerol

Connell and Sutherland (1969) first demonstrated the presence of a homologous series of phenolic ketones in ginger and the main pungent compounds in fresh ginger known as gingerols whereas the pungency of dry ginger mainly presence of shogaols. For example, [6]-shogaol is the dehydrated form of [6]-gingerol. The most abundant gingerol found in ginger is [6]-gingerol (Wang et al., 2011). Other gingerols with different chain lengths are also present in comparatively small quantities (Ali et al., 2008). Jolad et al., (2004) reported that they have identified 63 compounds on organically grown fresh ginger, 31 compounds from them had been previously reported as constituents of ginger and 20 were hitherto unknown compounds. The identified compounds included gingerols, shogaols, paradols, dihydroparadols, [3]-dihydroshogaols, acetyl derivatives of gingerols, gingerdiols, mono- and di-acetyl derivatives of gingerdiols, 1-dehydrogingerdiones, diarylheptanoids, and methyl ether derivatives of some of these compounds. In addition to [6]-gingerol, [4]-, [7]-, [8]-, and [10]-gingerol were identified. Figure 1 shows the chemical structures of the major gingerols and shogaol that are present in ginger. Masuda et al., (2004) suggested that the substituents on the alkyl chain of gingerol and related compounds might contribute to both radical scavenging effect and inhibitory effect on autoxidation of oils, while inhibitory effects against the AAPH-induced peroxidation of liposome was somewhat influenced by the alkyl chain length.

[6]-gingerol and [6]-shogaol are the two active components of ginger which produced a depressor response on blood pressure at lower doses (Suekawa et al., 1984).

B. Stability of 6-Gingerol

Wohlmuth et al., (2005) examined the stability of ethanolic extracts of ginger approximately 5 months at refrigerated (4 °C) temperature and observed that the concentration of [6]-gingerol did not change and this compound therefore appear to be stable in ethanolic solution under the refrigerated conditions. However, gingerols are thermally unstable and are converted into shogaols during the thermal processing (He et al., 1998). Degradation rates of [6]-gingerol to [6]-shogaol is pH dependent, with the greatest stability at pH 4, whereas at 100 ^{0}C and pH 1, the reversible degradation was relatively rapid (Bhattarai et al., 2001). Thermal degradation of gingerols to gingerone, shogaols, and related compounds was demonstrated by Jolad et al., (2004).

C. Pharmacokinetics, Bioavailability and Mammalian Metabolism of 6-Gingerol

A pharmacokinetic study was performed in rats by Ding et al., (1991) and they were able to achieve a quantitative analysis with high reproducibility for [6]-gingerol over the concentration range of 0.2-40 μg/mL and found that [6]-gingerol was rapidly cleared from plasma with a terminal half-life of 7.23 min and a total body clearance of 16.8 ml/min/kg subsequent bolus intravenous administration at a dose of 3 mg/kg. The reported serum protein binding of [6]-gingerol was 92.4% (Ding et al., 1991). The same group studied the kinetics in rats with experimental acute hepatic or renal failure (Naora et al.,

1992) and reported that there was no significant difference in either any pharmacokinetic parameters or plasma concentration–time curve between the control and nephrectomized rats suggesting that renal excretion does not contribute at all to the disappearance of [6]-gingerol from plasma in rats. In contrast, hepatic toxicity elevated the plasma concentration of [6]-gingerol at the terminal phase. Its elimination half-life increased significantly from 8.5 to 11.0 min, in rats with hepatic damage. The extent of [6]-gingerol bound to serum protein was more than 90% and was affected very slightly by the toxicity. These aspects indicate that [6]-gingerol is eliminated partly by the liver. Surh and Lee (1994) investigated the reductive metabolism of S-(+)-[6]-gingerol *in vitro* with phenobarbital-induced rat liver supernatant containing the NADPH-generating system. The reduction was shown to be stereo-specific. The ethyl acetate-extractable products were isolated and two metabolites were identified as diastereomers of [6]-gingerdiol by gas chromatography/mass spectrometry. The same authors have previously shown that [6]-shogaol, was reduced in rat liver *in vitro*. Recently, it has been reported that [6]-gingerol, when incubated with NADPH-fortified rat hepatic microsomes, gave rise to eight metabolites, which were tentatively identified by gas chromatography–mass spectrometry (GC–MS) analysis as two products of aromatic hydroxylation, as well as the diastereomers of two aliphatic hydroxylation products and the diastereomers of [6]-gingerdiol. Hepatic microsomes from rats and humans, fortified with UDPGA (urdine 5`-diphospho glucuronic acid), glucuronidated [6]-gingerol predominantly at the phenolic hydroxyl group, but small amounts of a second monoglucuronide involving the aliphatic hydroxyl group were also identified by liquid chromatography tandemmass spectrometry (LC-MS/MS) analysis. Human intestinal microsomes formed the phenolic glucuronide only (Pfeiffer et al., 2006). Supersomes containing human UGT1A1 and UGT1A3 exclusively generated the phenolic glucuronide, albeit with very low activities, whereas UGT1A9 catalyzed the specific formation of the alcoholic glucuronide, and UGT2B7 the predominant formation of the phenolic glucuronide, with high activities. This study revealed a rather complex metabolism of [6]-gingerol, which according to the authors, should be taken into consideration for the multiple biological activities of this compound (Pfeiffer et al., 2006). The metabolic fate of [6]-gingerol was investigated in rats by Nakazawa and Ohsawa (2002). The bile of rats that had been orally administered [6]-gingerol was shown by HPLC analysis to contain a major metabolite (S)-[6]-gingerol-40-O-β-glucuronide.

Although the metabolites derived from [6]-gingerol were not detected in the urine, the ethyl acetate extract of the urine, after enzymatic hydrolysis, was shown to contain six minor metabolites: vanillic acid, ferulic acid (S)-(+)-4-hydroxy-6-oxo-8-(4-hydroxy-3-methoxyphenyl)-octanoic acid, 4-(4-hydroxy-3-methoxyphenyl) butanoic acid, 9-hydroxy[6]-gingerol and (S)-(+)-[6]-gingerol. The total cumulative amount of the major metabolite excreted in the bile and of the six minor metabolites in the urine during 60 h after the oral administration of [6]-gingerol were approximately 48% and 16% of the dose, respectively. The excretion of the six minor metabolites in the urine decreased after gut sterilization, possibly suggesting the involvement of gut flora in the metabolism. On the other hand, incubation of [6]-gingerol with rat liver showed the presence of 9-hydroxy-[6]-gingerol, gingerdiol, and (S)-[6]-gingerol-40-*O*-β-glucuronide. These findings suggest that both the gut flora, as well as enzymes in the liver, play an important part in the metabolism of [6]-gingerol.

Zick et al., (2008) conducted a human clinical trial with [6]-gingerol, [8]-gingerol, [10]-gingerol, and [6]-shogaol, examining the pharmacokinetics and tolerability of these analytes and their conjugate metabolites. They found that the main pungent constituents of ginger root, [6]-gingerol, [8]-gingerol, [10]-gingerol, and [6]-shogaol, are quickly absorbed and detected in the serum as glucuronide and sulfate conjugates, with the majority detected as glucuronide metabolites. Yu et al., (2011) confirmed the same findings. These constituents, at concentrations normally found in ginger root (0.5%-2.5%), are detectable in the serum starting at a 1.0 g dose with the exception of [6]-gingerol, which is detectable at a 250 mg dose with maximum concentrations ranging from 0.1 μg/mL to 1.7 μg/mL. Yu et al., (2011) developed and validated a sensitive LC-MS/MS method for the simultaneous quantification of [6], [8], and [10]-gingerols and [6]-shogaol in the human plasma and they analyzed the pharmacokinetics of these ginger constituents and their metabolites. The half-lives ($T_{1/2}$) of [6], [8], and [10]-gingerols and [6]-shogaol and their metabolites are between 1 and 3 h in human plasma (Yu et al., 2011).

D. Antioxidant Properties

Recently, it has been shown that [6]-gingerol is endowed with strong antioxidant action both *in vivo* and *in vitro* (Kim et al., 2007). This makes it a very effective agent for prevention of ultra violet B (UVB)-induced reactive oxygen species production and COX-2 expression, and a possible therapeutic agent against UVB-induced skin disorders.

Masuda et al., (2004) indicated that the antioxidant activity of gingerols and related compounds might be due to not only radical scavenging activity of antioxidants but also their affinity of the antioxidants with substrates. Aeschbach et al., (1994) found that gingerol is good scavengers of peroxyl radicals generated by pulse radiolysis suggesting [6]-gingerol possess useful antioxidant properties and even may become important in the search for 'natural' replacements for 'synthetic' antioxidant food additives.

3. Biosynthesis in Plants

The biosynthesis of [6]-gingerol has been explicitly highlighted by Whiting and co-workers (Denniff et al., 1976; Macleod et al., 1979; Denniff et al., 1980). The biosynthetic pathway proposed by them indicated that phenylalanine is converted to ferulic acid through *p*-coumaric acid. As outlined in Figure 2, with the addition of reduction steps necessary to eliminate the double bond present in the *p*-coumaric acid-derived intermediate(s).

This reduction could occur prior to condensation or after condensation of the phenylpropanoid derived moiety with the CoA ester of the corresponding short chain aliphatic alcohol (Ramirez-Ahumada et al., 2006). Condensation of ferulic acid with malonate and hexanoate proceed to either by reacting with malonyl CoA to form β-ketoester and then to [6]-dehydrogingerdione or hexanoate reacting first with malonyl CoA and hydrolysis and following condensation with feruloyl-CoA leads to form 6-dehydrogingerdione. Both these pathways lead to [6]-dehydrogingerdione as the first intermediate with the complete C-skeleton of [6]-gingerol.

[6]-Gingerols could be produced through [6]-dehydrogingerdione. Enzymes in all of these proposed pathways would include one or more polyketide synthases, cytochrome p450 hydroxylases, and *S*-adenosyl-L-methionine-dependent *O*-methyltransferases. A study done by Ramirez-Ahumada et al., (2006) described the identification of such enzyme activities in ginger and turmeric tissues, and they provides the first direct evidence for enzymatic involvement of this phenylpropanoid pathway in the production of these compounds in plants.

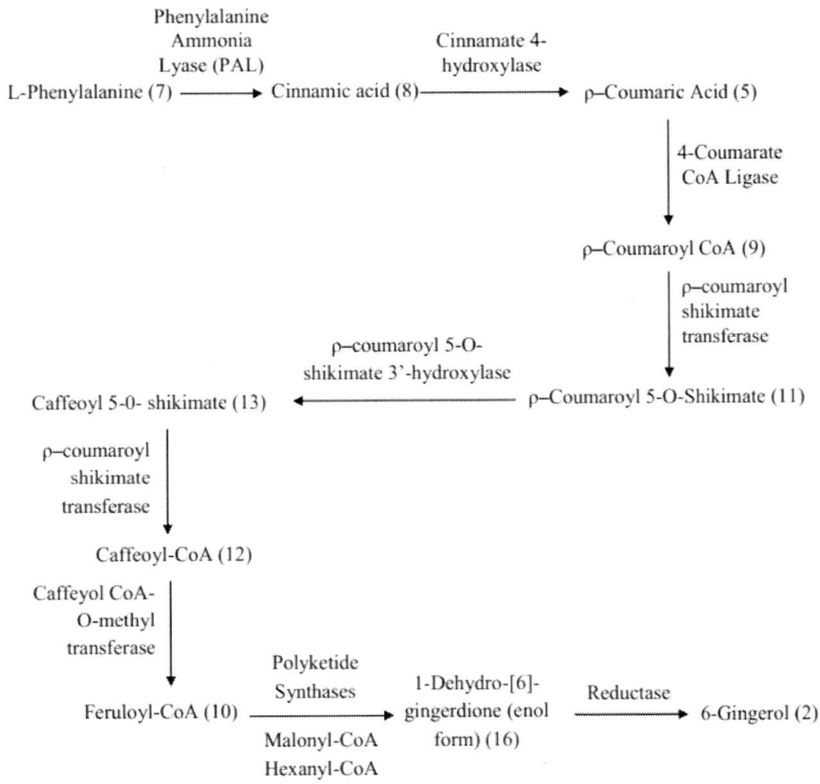

Figure 2. Proposed biosynthetic pathway of [6]-gingerol (adapted from Ramirez-Ahumada et al., 2006).

4. Analysis: Identification and Quantification

A. Thin-Layer Chromatography (TLC)

TLC has frequently been used for the separation and the quantitative or semi-quantitative analysis of natural compounds because of its advantages such as rapidity, easiness, and low cost. This method does not require complex instrumental equipment and it is more sensitive than paper chromatography (Guliyev et al., 2004). However, this method provides less quantitative information compared with HPLC– or GC–MS (Guliyev et al., 2004). A simple and rapid densitometric method has been developed by Melianata et al., (2009) for the determination of [6]-gingerol, [8]-gingerol, [10]-gingerol, and

[6]-shogaol in some commercial gingers. They extracted the samples four times with methanol and the solutions were spotted on pre-coated Lichrosphere Si 60F254 HPTLC plates, which were eluted with a mixture of toluene–ethyl acetate (3:1, v/v). Quantitative evaluation was done by measuring the absorbance reflectance of the analyte spots at $\lambda = 577$ nm after being sprayed with anisaldehyde-H_2SO_4 reagent. A similar type of research has been done by Connel and McLachlan (1972) and gingerols and other related compounds have been examined by TLC (silica gel). According to their findings, TLC gives only partial separation of the various homologous series of compounds, whereas good resolution is obtained with gas chromatography. However, they found compounds containing a β-hydroxy ketone grouping, *e.g.*, the gingerols, decompose to aliphatic aldehydes and zingerone under the conditions of gas chromatography. Furthermore, Chen et al., (1986) used the TLC to isolate gingerol compounds extracted from freeze-dried ginger using liquid carbon dioxide (600–700 p.s.i.), and fractionated into individual gingerol compounds with the use of preparative HPLC. Two homologous series, [6], [8], [10], [12], [14]-gingerols and methyl-[6]-, methyl-[8]-, methyl-[10]-, methyl-[12]-gingerols were identified by the combined results of HPLC retention time in analytical column; molecular ion determination of isolated gingerol compounds by fast atom bombardment-mass spectrometry; GC and GC-MS analyses of aldehydes and ketones formed from the thermal degradation of the corresponding gingerol compounds. This is the first report of the presence [14]-gingerol and gingerols with methyl side chains in ginger.

B. High-Performance Liquid Chromatography (HPLC)

HPLC is the most powerful and the most frequently used technique for natural compounds such as, saponins, carotenoids, sesquiterpenoids, etc. (Guliyev et al., 2004). It has also been used extensively for determination of pungent constituents in ginger. HPLC–MS and capillary electrophoresis methods have also been employed to determine phenolic compounds present in foods (He et al., 1997) including pungent constituents in ginger. There are many different LC–MS interfaces, each with certain selectivity and its own restrictions (Wolfender et al., 1994). In an Electrospray (ES) Interface the ions are formed from the liquid phase by ejection from shrinking charged droplets. This is more suitable for the analysis of compounds like gingerols as they are thermally unstable and decompose at high temperature during GC analysis. An improved HPLC separation of ginger constituents and the direct identification of the peaks in HPLC chromatograms from fresh ginger and ginger oleoresin by HPLC–UV–ES-MS analysis have been reported by He et al., (1998). According to their findings, seven compounds were positively identified as the major pungent constituents of ginger based on their UV spectra and comparison to data for the purified standards: [6]-gingerol and [6]-shogaol. The pungent compounds were assigned as [6]-gingerol, [8]-gingerol, [10]-gingerol, [6]-shogaol, [8]-shogaol, [10]-shogaol and [6]-gingediol. Another eight minor compounds were tentatively identified as gingerol analogues. Similarly, for the analysis of the major constituents of ginger ([6]-, [8]-, [10]-gingerol and [6]-shogaol) in dietary supplements, spices, teas and beverages containing the crude drug, an HPLC procedure has recently been published by Schwertner and Rios (2007).

Zick et al., (2010) developed a method to determine the main pungent ginger constituents, [6]-, [8]- and [10]-gingerols and [6]-shogaol in human plasma and quantitation was achieved using a reversed-phase C_{18} column using HPLC with electrochemical detection. They have found that the recovery of all four analytes was ≥ 99% for at 5.0 μg/mL and the lower limit of quantitation was 0.1 μg/mL except for [10]-gingerol which was 0.25 μg/mL. Currently, there is no analytical method for detecting pungent ginger constituents in human plasma. This HPLC method allows for the detection of all pungent constituents of ginger simultaneously in a relatively short run time of 25 minutes and therefore this method is useful for determining plasma levels of [6]-, [8]-,[10]-gingerol and [6]-shogaol in clinical trials. Gunathilake & Rupasinghe (2014a) have used Ultra Performance Liquid Chromatography (UPLC) coupled with ESI-MS and equipped with an acuity UPLC BEH C18 column to analyze the major phenolic bioactives of ginger according to the procedure reported by He et al., (1998).

C. High Speed Counter-Current Chromatography (HSCCC)

HSCCC is a kind of liquid–liquid partition chromatography without any solid matrix, which eliminates irreversible adsorption of samples on solid support in the conventional chromatographic column (Gu, et al., 2004). An optimized high speed countercurrent chromatographic (CCC) technique was used by Farthing and O'Neil (1990) for the isolation of [6]-, [8]- and [10]-gingerols, in quantities between 40 and 500 mg, from powdered root. Also they found that minor modifications to the procedure allowed the separation of

[4]-gingerol. The purity of the isolated gingerols has been assessed by proton nuclear magnetic resonance spectroscopy (NMR). According to their findings, of the 4 gingerols isolated only [8]-gingerol was shown to have a significant impurity (about 10%) with the purest being [6]-gingerol at >97%. It was concluded by them that the technique may be used for the preparation of samples of high purity suitable for use as analytical standards.

D. Nuclear Magnetic Resonance Spectroscopy (NMR)

Developments in the hyphenation of liquid chromatography and spectroscopy, particularly HPLC–MS and HPLC–NMR offer the potential for unknown peaks to be rapidly identified without the need for either extensive sample purification or synthetic standards (Wilson, 2000). As such these techniques are playing an increasingly important role in the study of natural products. For HPLC-NMR the use of superheated deuterium oxide as the eluent is advantageous compared to conventional HPLC organic–aqueous eluents as this would avoid the signals from the modifiers, which could otherwise interfere with the spectra of the analytes (Wilson, 2000). Catchpole et al., (2003) have analyzed acetone extracts of Australian and African ginger using NMR technique and they found that gingerol is the major component of NMR spectra of these ginger extracts which is about 30.4% and 20.9% w/w, respectively as [6]-gingerol. Furthermore, Kikuzaki et al., (1994) have isolated fourteen gingerol related compounds from ginger rhizomes and their structures were elucidated using NMR technique on the basis of chemical and spectroscopic evidence. The results of these studies demonstrate the applicability of NMR for the identification of the components of a natural product.

5. Potential Cardiovascular Effect of [6]-Gingerol - *In Vitro*, *In Vivo* and Human Clinical Studies

A. Effect on Atherosclerosis and Lipid Metabolism

The inhibitory actions of [6]-gingerol against low density lipo-protein (LDL) oxidation were studied *in vitro* by Lam et al., (2007) and found that [6]-

gingerol exhibit strong inhibition against lipid peroxidation in LDL induced by 2,2-azobis (2-amidinopropane) hydrochloride (AAPH) and hemin. IC_{50} values (μM) of [6]-gingerol for inhibition of AAPH-induced lipid peroxidation in LDL, inhibition of hemin-induced lipid peroxidation in LDL, inhibition of AAPH-induced hemolysis and inhibition of lipid peroxidation of erythrocyte membranes were 19.1, 0.054, 95.3 and 20.7, respectively (Lam et al., 2007). Similarly, in an in vitro study by Gunathilake & Rupasinghe (2014a), have reported that pure phenolic bioactives of ginger, including [6]-gingerol were strong inhibitors of copper-induced human LDL oxidation in vitro.

The use of gingerols or gingerdiol derivatives for lowering plasma cholesterol, inhibiting the progression of atherosclerosis and inhibiting the peroxidation of LDL was claimed by Mao and King (1993). In an *in vivo* study with mice showed that oral administration of [6]-gingerol significantly ($p < 0.05$) reduces the plasma triglycerides, total cholesterol, free fatty acid, LDL-cholesterol and plasma insulin concentration (Singh et al., 2009). Similarly, Gunathilake et al., (2013a) reported that a functional beverage incorporated with [6]-gingerol-rich extract have shown a hypo-cholesterolaemic effect in spontaneously hypertensive rats (SHR). In addition, [6]-gingerol significantly ($p < 0.05$) reduces the content of hydrogen peroxide or suppresses the reactive oxygen species generation and restores the enzyme activity of catalase, glutathione peroxidase and superoxide dismutase in db/db mice (Singh et al., 2009). Further, Saravanan et al (2014) have reported that the dose of 75 mg kg^{-1} of gingerol was more pronounced in suppressing the obesity induced by high fat diet including plasma and tissue fat. In an another study, It was reported that beneficial modification of the lipoprotein profile by dietary gingerol-enriched extract to enhance the excretion of fecal cholesterol and bile acids via up-regulation of hepatic cholesterol-7α-hydroxylase and down-regulation of mRNA of intestinal Niemann–Pick C1-like 1 protein, acyl CoA cholesterol acyltransferase 2 and microsomal triacylglycerol transport protein (Lei et al., 2014).

These findings suggest that [6]-gingerol exhibits a significant potential as lipid lowering and antioxidant effects, therefore, Gunathilake et al., (2013a) suggested that the water extracts of ginger can be incorporated into fruit-based functional beverages designed for cardio-protection. Gunathilake & Rupasinghe (2014b) have also described an ultrasonication based extraction method to prepare [6]-gingerol-rich extract for functional formulations.

B. Fibrinolytic Activity

Inhibition or deficiency of the factors involved in fibrinolytic activity might disturb the hemostatic balance and allow excessive fibrin deposition leading to situations such as hypertension, and hypercholesterolemia. It is also possible that disturbance in the coagulation-fibrinolytic system may result in the development of thrombosis and ischemia (Banerjee and Maulik, 2002). Effect of supplementation of gingerol-rich ginger powder on fibrinolytic activity of healthy individuals given with high-fat diet has been studied by Varma and Bordia (2001). It was found that addition of gingerol-rich ginger powder along with the fat not only prevented the fall in fibrinolytic activity but actually increased it significantly. This fibrinolytic enhancing property of gingerol is a further addition to the therapeutic potential of gingerol towards the cardiovascular diseases (Varma and Bordia, 2001).

C. Platelet Aggregation

Gingerols, the active components of ginger, represent a potential new class of platelet activation inhibitors in human (Koo et al., 2001). In an *in vitro* study, ability of a series of synthetic gingerols and related phenylalkanol analogues (G1–G7) to inhibit human platelet activation was compared with aspirin (Nurtjahja-Tjendraputra et al., 2003), by measuring their effects on arachidonic acid (AA)-induced platelet serotonin release and aggregation. This study revealed that the IC_{50} for inhibition of AA-induced serotonin release by [6]-gingerol (45.3-82.6 mM) is significantly higher than aspirin (23.4 ± 3.6 mM). The mechanism underlying inhibition of the AA-induced platelet release reaction and aggregation by gingerol and related compounds may be via an effect on cyclooxygenase (COX) activity in platelets because these compounds potently inhibited COX activity in rat basophilic leukemia (RBL-2H3) cells (Nurtjahja-Tjendraputra et al., 2003). These results provide a basis for the design of more potent synthetic gingerol analogues, with similar potencies to aspirin, as platelet activation inhibitors with potential value in cardiovascular disease (Koo et al., 2001). In another *in vitro* study, Hong et al., (2008) have indicated that [6]-gingerol, [8]-gingerol, [6]-shogaol and [10]-gingerol had an anti-platelet aggregation activity which was done using chicken thrombocyte extract and HPLC and also they confirmed these activities using platelet aggregation *in vivo*. Furthermore, gingerol inhibited the aggregation and release reaction of rabbit washed platelets induced by arachidonic acid and collagen, but not those induced by platelet-activating factor and thrombin in a concentration dependently manner and they indicated that the antiplatelet action of gingerol is mainly due to the inhibition of thromboxane formation (Guh et al., 1995). The above pharmacological evidence has suggested that ginger constituents and related substances could be potential antiplatelet substances, like aspirin, without causing adverse events.

D. Blood Pressure Lowering Effect

In addition to the ginger extracts, some of ginger pure constituents, [6]-gingerol and [6]-shogaol have been studied for their effects on blood pressure in laboratory animals (Suekawa et al., 1984) where both were found to produce a depressant effect, at lower doses, and a tri-phasic effect (consisting of an initial hypotensive followed by a sharp hypertensive and then a delayed hypotensive effect), at the higher doses, in rats under anaesthesia. Later, reports revealed that the peripheral pressor effect of [6]-shogaol in rats is caused by release of a peptide-like substance from the sympathetic nerve endings (Suekawa et al., 1986). Some of the known pungent constituents of ginger including [6]-gingerol tested for vasodilator activity in the endothelium-intact rat aorta and it was found that these gingerols exhibited more vasodilator effect on the phenylephrine (PE) and high K^+-induced contractions (Thorin et al., 1998). The observed vasodilator effect of gingerols was insensitive to atropine pretreatment but considerable blockade was observed in the presence of an NO synthase inhibitor (Thorin et al., 1998). [6]-Gingerol was also able to relax the high K^+-induced contractions indicating the co-existence of a Ca^{++} antagonist-type component (Bolton, 1979). 6-Gingerol has been reported for an inhibitory response on the spontaneous contractions and Ca^{++} spikes in isolated portal veins of mice (Kimura et al.,1988) thus supporting the conclusion of a Ca^{++} antagonist action. The relatively simple phenols such as gingerol are activators of cardiac sarcoplasmic reticulum calcium pumping ATPase (Kobayashi et al., 1987, 1988) and this enzyme is mainly responsible for the rapid removal of Ca^{++} ions from the cytosol which allows efficient relaxation of cardiac muscle cells (Ghisalberti et al., 1998). In a study with healthy human subjects, it was reported that the consumption of ginger extract has a blood pressure lowering effect in a dose-dependent manner (Ojulari et al., 2014).

Conclusion

6-Gingerol is a unique group of phenolic compounds that have demonstrated a multiple of pharmacological effects including anti-atherosclerotic, antihypertensive, antiplatelet-aggregation effects and fibrinolytic activity. Pharmacokinetic studies *in vivo* have also confirmed that gingerols are bioavailable and reviewed findings suggest that both the gut flora, as well as enzymes in the liver, play an important part in the metabolism of [6]-gingerol. The biosynthesis of 6-gingerol has been highlighted by Whiting and coworkers and enzymes in all of these proposed pathways would include polyketide synthase, cytochrome p450 hydroxylases and S-adenosyl-L-methionine dependent *O*-methyltransferases. Reviewed *in vivo* and *in vitro* studies revealed that 6-gingerol exhibits a significant potential as a lipid lowering and LDL oxidation inhibiting agent. In a clinical study, it was found that gingerol increased the fibrinolytic activity of healthy individuals given with high fat diet. Pharmalogical evidence indicated that [6]-ginegrols could be potential antiplatelet substance and the effect is comparable with aspirin. Furthermore, [6]-gingerol exhibited vasodilator activity and activate the cardiac sarcoplasmic reticulum calcium pumping ATPase which allows efficient relaxation of cardiac muscle cells. Consequently, many types of analytical methods have been developed for the identification and quantification of [6]-gingerol in raw materials and preparations. In particular, analytical HPLC combined with various interfaces, and/or MS detection has shown to be useful for the analysis of nearly all types of gingerols. So far, focus has been primarily on the quantification of major bioactives in rhizome of ginger. Therefore, many interesting pharmacological effects of gingerols are yet to be discovered from other parts of the plant. The pharmacological effects of 6-gingerol and other gingerols are required to be further investigated in relation to other chronic disorders.

References

Aeschbach, R; J. Löliger; Scott, B.C.; Murcia, A.; Butler, J.; Halliwell, B; Aruoma, O.I. Antioxidant actions of thymol, carvacrol, 6-gingerol, zingerone and hydroxytyrosol. *Food and Chem. Toxicol.* 1994, *32(1)*, 31-36.

Ahmed, R.S.; Seth, V.; Banerjee, B.D. Influence of dietary ginger (*Zingiber officinale*) on antioxidant defense system in rat: Comparison with ascorbic acid. *Indian J of Experi. Biology*. 2000, *38(6),* 604-606.

Ali, B. H. Blunden, G. Tanira, M.O., Nemmar, A. Some physico-chemical, pharmacological and toxicological properties of ginger (*Zingerber officinale*)-a review. *Food and Chem. Toxico.* 2008, *46,* 409-410.

Banerjee, S.K.; Maulik, S.K. Effect of garlic on cardiovascular disorders: a review. *Nutri. Journal.* 2002, *1(4).*

Bhattarai, S.; Tran, V. H.; Duke, C. C. The stability of gingerol and shogaol in aqueous solution. *J. Pharm. Sci.* 2001, *90*, 1658–1664.

Bode, A. M.; Ma, W. Y.; Surh, Y. J.; Dong, Z. Inhibition of epidermal growth factor-induced cell transformation and activator protein 1 activation by [6]-gingerol. *Cancer Res.* 2001, *61*, 850–853.

Bolton, T. B. Mechanism of action of transmitters and other substances on smooth muscles. *Physiol. Rev.*1979, *59*, 606–718.

Catchpole, O. J.; Grey, J. B.; Perry, N. B.; Burgess, E. J.; Redmond, W.A.; Porter, N.G. Extraction of Chili, Black Pepper, and Ginger with Near-Critical CO2, Propane, and Dimethyl Ether: Analysis of the Extracts by Quantitative Nuclear Magnetic Resonance *J. Agric. Food Chem.* 2003, *51,* 4853-4860.

Chen, C.; Rosen, R.T.; Ho, C. Chromatographic analyses of gingerol compounds in ginger (*Zingiber officinale* roscoe) extracted by liquid carbon dioxide. *J. of Chromatography A*, 1986, *360,* pp.163-173.

Connell, D.W.; McLachlan, R. Natural pungent compounds: examination of gingerols, shogaols, paradols and related compounds by thin-layer and gas chromatography. *J. Chromatogr.* 1972, *67*, 29–35.

Connell, D.W.; Sutherland, M.D. A re-examination of gingerol, shogaol, and zingerone, the pungent principles of ginger (*Zingiber officinale* Roscoe). *Australian Journal of Chemistry.*1969, *22(5),* 1033 – 1043.

Denniff, P.; Macleod, I.; Whiting. D.W. Biosynthesis of [6]-gingerol, pungent principle of *Zingiber officinale J. Chem. Soc., Chem. Commun.* 1976, 711-712.

Denniff, P.; Macleod, I.; Whiting. D.W. Studies in the Biosynthesis of [6]-Gingerol, Pungent Principle of Ginger *(Zingiber officinale. J. Chem. Soc., Perkin Trans. 1*. 1980, 2637-2644.

Ding, G. H.; Naora, K.; Hayashibara, M.; Katagiri, Y.; Kano, Y.; Iwamoto, K. Pharmacokinetics of [6]-gingerol after intravenous administration in rats. *Chem. Pharm. Bull. (Tokyo)*. 1991, *39*, 1612–1614.

Farthing, J. E.; O'Neill, M. J. Isolation of gingerols from powdered root ginger by countercurrent chromatography. *J. of Liquid Chromatogra.* 1990, *13(5)* pp. 941-950.

Ficker, C.; Smith, M. L.; Akpagana, K.; Gbeassor, M.; Zhang, J.; Durst, T.; et al., Bioassay-guided isolation and identification of antifungal compounds from ginger. *Phytotherapy Res.* 2003, *17*, 897–902.

Ghayur, M. N.; Gilani, A. H. Ginger lowers blood pressure through blockade of voltage-dependent calcium channels. *J. Cardiovasc.Pharmacol.* 2005, *45*, 74–80.

Ghayur, M. N.; Gilani, A. H.; Afridi, M. B.; Houghton, P. J. Cardiovascular effects of ginger aqueous extract and its phenolic constituents are mediated through multiple pathways. *Vascul. Pharmacol.* 2005, *43*, 234–241.

Ghisalberti, E. L.; Pennacchio, M.; Alexander, E. Survey of secondary plant metabolites with cardiovascular activity. *Pharm. Biology.* 1998, *36(4)*, 237–279.

Gu, M.; Ouyang, F.; Su, Z. Comparison of high-speed counter-current chromatography and high-performance liquid chromatography on fingerprinting of Chinese traditional medicine. *J. of Chromatogra. A.* 2004, *(1022)*, pp 139–144.

Guh, F.; Ko, F.; Jong; T.; Teng. C. Antiplatelet effect of gingerol isolated from Zingiber officinale. *J. of Pharmacy and Pharmacology.* 1995, *47(4)*, 329–332.

Gupta, S. K. and Sharma, A. Medicinal properties of *Zingiber officinale* Roscoe - A Review, *IOSR Journal of Pharmacy and Biological Sciences,* 2014, *9(5), 124-129.*

Guliyev VB, Gul M, Yildirim A. *Hippophae rhamnoides* L.: chromatographic methods to determine chemical composition, use in traditional medicine and pharmacological effects, *J. Chromatogr B*, 2004, *812* (1-2),291–307.

Gunathilake K.D.P.P., Pitts, N., Rupasinghe, H. P. V. Formulation and characterization of a bioactives-enriched fruit beverage designed for cardio-protection. *Food Research International*, 2013(a), *52(2)*, 535-541.

Gunathilake K.D.P.P., Wang, Y., Rupasinghe, H. P. V. Evaluation of cardio-protective properties of functional beverage using an animal model of spontaneously hypertensive rats. *Journal of Functional Foods*, 2013(b), *5,* 1392-1401.

Gunathilake K.D.P.P., Rupasinghe, H. P. V. Inhibition of human low density lipoprotein oxidation in vitro by ginger extracts. Journal of Medicinal Foods, 2014(a), *17 (4)*, 424-431.

Gunathilake K.D.P.P., Rupasinghe, H. P. V. Optimization of water based-extraction methods for the preparation of bioactive rich ginger extract using response surface methodology. *European Journal of Medicinal Plants*, 2014(b), *4(8).*

He, X. G.; Bernart, M. W.; Lian, L.-S.; Lin, L.-Z. High performance liquid chromatography-electrospray mass spectrometric analysis of pungent constituents of ginger. *J. Chromatogr.* 1998, *796*, 327-334.

He, X.G.; Lian, L, Z.; Lin, L.Z.; Bernart, M. Liquid chromatography–electrospray mass spectrometric analysis of curcuminoids and sesquiterpenoids in turmeric (*Curcuma longa*). *J. Chromatogr. A.* 1997. *791 (127).*

Hibino, T.; Yuzurihara, M.; Terawaki, K.; Kanno, H.; Kase, Y.; Takeda, A. Goshuyuto, a traditional Japanese medicine for migraine, inhibits platelet aggregation in guinea-pig whole blood. *J. of Pharmacological Sci.* 2008, *108,* 89–94.

Hong, N.; Lan-zhen, M.; Hui, Z.; Jian-yu, Z.; Zhen, Y.; Xue-song, H. Analysis of anti-platelet aggregation components of Rhizoma Zingiberis using chicken thrombocyte extract and high performance liquid chromatography. *Chinese Medic. J.* 2008, 121(13), 1226.

Ippoushi, K.; Azuma, K.; Ito, H.; Horie, H.; Higashio, H. [6]-Gingerol inhibits nitric oxide synthesis in activated J774.1 mouse macrophages and prevents peroxynitrite-induced oxidation and nitration reactions. ***Life Sci.*** 2003, *73(26),* 3427-3437.

Jolad, S. D.; Lantz, R. C.; Solyon, A. M.; Chen, G. J.; Bates, R. B.; Timmermann, B. N. Fresh organically grown ginger (Zingiber officinale): composition and effects on LPS-induced PGE2 production. *Phytochemistry.* 2004, *65*, 1937–1954.

Jolad, S. D.; Lantz, R.C.; Chen, G.J.; Bates, R.B.; Timmermann, B.N. commercially processed dry ginger (Zingiber officinale): composition and effects on LPS-stimulated PGE2 production. *Phytochemistry.* 2005, *66,* 1614–1635.

Katiyar, S. K.; Agarwal, R.; Mukhta, H. Inhibition of tumor promotion inmSENCAR mouse skin by ethanol extract of Zingiber officinale rhizome. *Cancer Res.* 1996, *56*, 1023–1030.

Kikuzaki, H.; Kawasaki, Y.; Nakatani, N. Structure of Antioxidative Compounds in Ginger. *Food Phytochem. for Cancer Prevention II* Chapter 24, *ACS Symposium Series*, American. Chemical Society. 1994, 547, 237-243.

Kim, J. K.; Kim, Y.; Na, K. M.; Surh, Y. J.; Kim, T. Y. [6]-Gingerol prevents UVB-induced ROS production and COX-2 expression in vitro and in vivo. *Free Radi. Res.* 2007, *41*, 603–614.

Kim, S. O.; Chun, K. S.; Kundu, J. K.; Surh, Y. J. Inhibitory effects of [6]-gingerol on PMA-induced COX-2 expression and activation of NF-kappaB and p38 MAPK in mouse skin. *BioFactors.* 2004, *21*, 27–31.

Kim, S. O.; Kundu, J. K.; Shin, Y. K.; Park, J. H.; Cho, M. H.; Kim, T. Y. et al., [6]-Gingerol inhibits COX-2 expression by blocking the activation of p38 MAP kinase and NF-kappaB in phorbol ester-stimulated mouse skin. *Oncogene.* 2005, *24*, 2558–2567.

Kimura, I.; Pancho, L. R.; Shiori, T.; Kimura, M. Suppression of spontaneous calcium spikes and contraction in isolated portal veins of mice by gingerols and chemically related compounds. *Jpn. J. Pharmacol.*1988, *48*, 257–262.

Kobayashi M; Ishida Y.; Shoji N; Ohimuzi Y. Cardiotonic effect of [8]-gingerol, an activator of calciumpumping adenosine triphosphatase of sarcoplasmic reticulum in guinea pig atrial muscle. *J. Pharmacol Exp Ther.* 1988, *246,* 667–673.

Kobayashi M; Shoji N.; Ohimuzi Y. Gingerol, a novel cardiotonic agent, activates the Ca21-pumping ATPase in skeletal and cardiac sarcoplasmic reticulum. *Biochem Biophys Acta* .1987, *903,* 96–102.

Koo, K. L. K.; Ammit, A. J.; Tran, V. H.; Duke, C. C.; Roufogalis, B. D. Gingerols and related analogues inhibit arachidonic acid-induced human platelet serotonin release and aggregation. *Thrombosis Res.* 2001, *103*, 387–397.

Lam, R. Y.; Woo, A. Y.; Leung, P. S.; Cheng, C. H. Antioxidant actions of phenolic compounds found in dietary plants on low-density lipoprotein and erythrocytes in vitro. *J. of the Ameri. Col. of Nutri.* 2007, *26*, 233–242.

Langner, E.; Greifenberg, S.; Gruenwald, J. Ginger: history and use. *Adv. Ther.* 1998, *15*, 25– 44.

Lei, L, Liu, Y, Wang, X., Jiao, R., Ying Ma, K., Li, Y.M., Wang, L., Man, S.M., Sang, S., Huang, Y. and Chen, Z. Plasma Cholesterol-Lowering Activity of Gingerol- and Shogaol-Enriched Extract Is Mediated by Increasing Sterol Excretion. *J. Agric. Food Chem.*, 2014, *62* (43), pp 10515–10521.

Li, X., H., McGrath K.C., Tran, V.H. et al., Attenuation of proinflammatory responses by S-[6]-gingerol via inhibition of ROS/NF-Kappa B/COX2 activation in HuH7 cells. 2013, Evidence based complementary and Alternative Medicine.

Macleod, I.; Whiting. D.W. Stages in the biosynthesis of [6]-gingerol in *zingiber Officinale J. Chem. Soc., Chem. Commun.* 1979, 1152-1153.

Mao, S. J. T.; King, C. H. R. Gingerol derivatives as antioxidants. *Current Opinion in Therap. Patents.* 1993, 3(5), 649-650.

Masuda, Y.; Kikuzaki, H.; Hisamoto, M.; Nakatani, N. Antioxidant properties of gingerol related compounds from ginger. *BioFactors*, 2004, *21*, 293–296.

Melianita, F., With a, J., Arifin, S., Kartiasari, W.F., Indrayanto, G. Simultaneous densitometric determination of 6-gingerol, 8-gingerol, 10-gingerol and 6-shogaol in some commercial gingers. *J. Liq. Chromatogr. Rel. Technol*, 2009, 32: 567-577.

Minghetti, P.; Sosa, S.; Cilurzo, F.; Casiraghi, A.; Alberti, E.; Tubaro, A. Evaluation of the topical anti-inflammatory activity of ginger dry extracts from solutions and plasters. *Planta Medica*. 2007, *73*, 1525–1530.

Nakazawa, T.; Ohsawa, K. Metabolism of [6]-gingerol in rats. *Life Sci.* 2002, *70*, 2165–2175.

Naora, K.; Ding, G.; Hayashibara, M.; Katagiri, Y.; Kano, Y.; Iwamoto, K. Pharmacokinetics of [6]-gingerol after intravenous administration in rats with acute renal or hepatic failure. *Chem. Pharm. Bull. (Tokyo).* 1992, *40*, 1295–1298.

Nie, H.; Meng, L. Z.; Zhang, H.; Zhang, J. Y.; Yin, Z.; Huang, X. S. Analysis of anti-platelet aggregation components of Rhizoma Zingiberis using chicken thrombocyte extract and high performance liquid chromatography. *Chinese Med. J.* 2008, *121*, 1226–1229.

Nurtjahja-Tjendraputra E; Ammit, A. J.; Roufogalis B. D.; Tran V. H; Duke C. C. Effective anti-platelet and COX-1 enzyme inhibitors from pungent constituents of ginger. *Thrombosis Resea*. 2003, *111*, 259–265.

Ojulari, L. S., Olatubosun, O. T., Okesina, K. B., and Owoyele, B. V. The Effect of Zingiber Officinale (Ginger) Extract on Blood Pressure and Heart Rate in Healthy Humans, *IOSR Journal of Dental and Medical Sciences,* 2014, *13(10),* 76-78.

Pfeiffer, E.; Heuschmid, F.F.; Kranz, S.; Metzler, M. Microsomal hydroxylation and glucuronidation of [6]-gingerol. *J. Agric. Food Chem.* 2006, *54*, 8769–8774.

Ramirez-Ahumada M.D.C.; Timmermann, B.N; Gang, D.R. Biosynthesis of curcuminoids and gingerols in turmeric (*Curcuma longa*) and ginger (*Zingiber officinale*): Identification of curcuminoid synthase and hydroxycinnamoyl-CoA thioesterases. *Phytochem.* 2006, *67(18)*, 2017-2029.

Saravanan, G., Ponmurugan, P., Deepa, M. A. and Senthilkumar, B. Anti-obesity action of gingerol: effect on lipid profile, insulin, leptin, amylase and lipase in male obese rats induced by a high-fat diet. 2014, *Journal of the Science of Food and Agriculture*, 2014, *94 (14)*, 2972–2977.

Schwertner, H.A.; Rios, C. High-performance liquid chromatography analysis of 6-gingerol, 8-gingerol, 10 gingerol and 6- shogaol in ginger-containing dietary supplements, spices, teas and beverages. *J. Chromatogr. B,* 2007, *856*, 41-47.

Shukla, Y.; Singh, M. Cancer preventive properties of ginger: A brief review. Food and Chem Toxico. 2007, *45*, 683–690.

Singh, A. B.; Singh, A. N.; Maurya, R.; Srivastava, A. K. Anti-hyperglycaemic, lipid lowering and anti-oxidant properties of [6]-gingerol in db/db mice. *Inter. J. of Medicine and Medical Sci.* 2009, 1(12), 536-544.

Suekawa, M.; Aburada, M.; Hosoya, E. Pharmacological studies on ginger: II. Pressor action of 6-shogaol in anaesthetized rats, or hindquarters, tail and mesenteric beds of rats. *J. Pharmacobio-dyn.* 1986. *9*, 842– 852.

Suekawa, M.; Ishige, A.; Yuasa, K.; Sudo, K.; Aburada, M.; Hosoya, E. Pharmacological studies on ginger: I. Pharmacological actions of pungent constituents, 6-gingerol and 6-shogaol. *J. Pharmacobio-dyn.* 1984, *7*, 836– 848.

Surh, Y. J.; Lee, S.S. Enzymic reduction of gingerol, a major pungent principle of ginger, in the cell-free preparation of rat liver. *Life Sci.* 1994, *54*, 321–326.

Thorin, E.; Huang, P.L.; Fishman, M.C.; Bevan, J.A. Nitric oxide inhibits alpha2-adrenoceptor-mediated endothelium-dependent vasodilation. *Circ. Res.* 1998, *82*, 1323– 1329.

Verma, S. K.; Bordia, A. Ginger, fat and fibrinolysis. *Indian J. of Medi. Sci.* 2001, *55 (2)*, 83-86.

Wang, X.; Zheng, Z.; Guo, X; Yuan, J.; Zheng, C. Preparative separation of gingerols from Zingiber officinale by high-speed counter-current chromatography using stepwise elution. *Food Chem.* 2011, *125*, 1476–1480.

Wilson, I. D. Multiple hyphenation of liquid chromatography with nuclear magnetic resonance spectroscopy, mass spectrometry and beyond. *J. of Chromatogr.* A. 2000, *892(1-2)*, 315-327.

Wohlmuth, H.; Leach, D. N.; Smith, M. K.; Myers, S. P. Gingerol content of diploid and tetraploid clones of ginger (Zingiber officinale Roscoe). *J. Agric. Food Chem.* 2005, *53*, 5772–5778.

Wolfender, J. L.; Hostettmann, K.; Arnason, J. T.; Mata, R.; Romeo, J. T (Eds.), Recent Advances in Phytochemistry, vol. 29, Phytochemistry of Medicinal Plants, Plenum Press, NewYork, 1994, pp. 237–243.

Yu, Y.; Zick, S.; Li, X. ; Zou, P. ; Wright, B. ; Sun, D. Examination of the pharmacokinetics of active ingredients of ginger in humans. *AAPS Journal.* 2011, *13(3),* 417-426.

Zick, S. M. ; Djuric, Z.; Ruffin, M. T. ; Litzinger, A. J. ; Normolle, D. P. ; Alrawi, S. ; Feng, M. R.; Brenner, D. E. Pharmacokinetics of 6-gingerol, 8-gingerol, 10-gingerol, and 6-shogaol and conjugate metabolites in healthyhuman subjects. *Cancer Epidem. Biomarkers and Preven.* 2008, *17(8)*, 1930-1936.

Zick, S. M.; Ruffin, M. T. ; Djuric, Z. ; Normolle, D.; Brenner, D. E. Quantitation of 6-, 8- and 10-gingerols and 6-shogaol in human plasma by high performance liquid chromatography with electrochemical detection. *Intern J. of Biomed Sci.* 2010, *6(3),* 233-240.

In: Ginger
Editor: Janine L. Perry

ISBN: 978-1-63482-020-2

Chapter 6

HYDRODISTILLATION: HEADSPACE SOLVENT MICROEXTRACTION AND CHEMICAL COMPOSITION OF KOREAN GINGER BY GAS CHROMATOGRAPHY AND MASS SPECTROMETRY

Dinesh C. Bilehal[1]* and Yong H. Kim[2]†
[1]Department of Chemistry, Reva Institute of Technology and Management, Yalhanka, Bangalore India
[2]Department of Biomedical Laboratory Science, Inje University, Kimhae, Gyeongnam, South Korea

ABSTRACT

In this study, a gas chromatography–mass spectrometry method in EI mode is developed for the analysis of dried Korean ginger. Hydro distillation–headspace solvent microextraction with polar and non-polar solvents is used. Forty-nine compounds are separated and identified. Some of the ginger compounds partially or completely were thermally decomposed. Some of these decomposition products likely produced when ginger is used in cooking at high temperatures and subsequently eaten. The major compounds in the rhizome identified are α-zingiberene,

* E-mail: drbilehal@gmail.com.
† E-mail: mlskimyh@inje.ac.kr.

curcumene, camphene, β-phellandrene, (E)-citral, α-farnesene, β-bisabolene, β-sesquiphellandrene, zingerone, and [6]-gingerol. This method will be useful for rapid screening purpose of plant samples for finding of high quality ginger under the plant breeding program, genotypes assessment, and also export quality of ginger species.

Keywords: Korean Ginger, Hydrodistillation–Headspace Solvent Microextraction, Gas Chromatography–Mass, Spectrometry, Gingerol, Curcumene

INTRODUCTION

Ginger (Zingiber officinale Roscoe, Zingiberacae) is a medicinal plant and also culinary spice that has been widely used in Ayurvedic (Sivarajan and Balachandran 1994), Chinese, and Tibb-Unani herbal medicines all over the world for a wide array of ailments. Currently, there is a renewed interest in ginger, and several scientific investigations aimed at isolation, identification of active constituents of ginger, and scientific verification of its pharmacological actions are in progress. Ginger has excellent antioxidant properties. Antioxidants are increasingly linked to the prevention of certain cancers (Kikuzaki et al. 1994; Park et al. 1998). Ginger has a known influence on functions such as wound healing, inflammation, and platelet aggregation and is involved in conditions such as arteriosclerosis (Srivasta 1986; Sankawa 1987; Kiuchi et al. 1992).

Ginger is on the FDA's generally recognized as safe list, though it does interact with some medications. It is considered a safe herbal medicine with only few and insignificant side effects. Ginger is contraindicated in people suffering from gallstones as the herb promotes the release of bile from the gallbladder. Ginger may also decrease joint pain from arthritis, though studies on this have been inconsistent, and may have blood thinning and cholesterol lowering properties (Tanabe et al. 1993) that may make it useful for treating heart disease. In laboratory animals, the gingerols increase the motility of the gastrointestinal tract (Yamahara et al. 1990) and have analgesic, sedative, antipyretic, and antibacterial properties. It has also been investigated for its gastroprotectant and antiulcer activity (Yamahara et al. 1988, 1992; Yoshikawa et al. 1994). Today, ginger root is widely used as a digestive aid for mild stomach upset and is commonly recommended by health care professionals to help prevent or treat nausea and vomiting associated with motion sickness and pregnancy.

Ginger does not reproduce by seed, but is clonally propagated via rhizome division and replanting. The contents in ginger from different places, in fact likely to possess different properties, not only in flavor and pungency, but also in potential bioactivity and health benefits. Variation in the amount of the constituent in ginger with the geographic areas, from one season to another, with different plant parts and morphology, and also with climatic and ecologic conditions. Earlier the Chinese and Japanese ginger analysis is reported and as per our knowledge there is no report available with Korean ginger. So we have tried to analyze the Korean ginger in this work.

Many compounds in a plant extract will not ionize optimally, or at all, by LC/MS, under the conditions employed in a single analytical run. Currently, metabolic profiling by LC/MS is more suited to groups of compounds, such as alkaloids, which ionize similarly under given conditions. In complex mixtures such as plant extracts, some compounds will preferentially form positive ions, others negative ions and some will be difficult to ionize under fixed conditions.

So, we have used gas chromatography–mass spectrometry (GC-MS) as analytical method for the evaluation of ginger and its constituents. Various analytical techniques employing chromatographic methods such as GLC and GC in conjunction with mass spectroscopy have been used to analyze pungent components in ginger by derivatizing the ginger extract to improve their volatility, stability, and separation (Masada et al. 1973; Clark et al. 1977; Harvey 1981; Masada et al. 1974). In present work, GC-MS analysis of the underivatized active fractions provided high resolution of the 49 components. In this work, ginger was extracted with polar and non-polar solvents, i.e., chloroform dichloromethane, ethanol, benzene, and hexane. The dichloromethane extract has exhibited better chromatogram in GC-MS analysis. So we report the use of GC-MS in accomplishing this effort.

Material and Methods

Fresh ginger (Z. officinale) was purchased from a local supermarket. The ginger rhizomes were stored under refrigerated conditions and washed thoroughly prior to use. Washed ginger was sliced to small pieces and dried in the oven at 60 °C for about 1 h. The unpeeled ginger is used for solvent extraction, since peeled ginger loses much of its essential oil content. The ginger sample was used for extraction within 30 min after drying.

Hydrodistillation–Headspace Solvent Microextraction

Hydrodistillation with concurrent headspace solvent microextraction (HD-HSME) was performed by using the apparatus shown in Figure 1. A 100-ml round-bottom flask containing 10 g of the ginger and 70 ml of water was heated at 100°C by a mantle. The Hamilton syringe was rinsed and primed at least seven times with the different solvents such as benzene, hexane, chloroform, dichloromethane, and ethanol solution. The syringe plunger was depressed and a microdrop of extracting solvent (benzene, hexane, chloroform, dichloromethane, and ethanol solution) was suspended from the needle tip. After 20 min of time, the plunger was withdrawn and the microdrop was retracted carefully back into the syringe. The needle was removed from the headspace and its contents were injected into the GC-MS system. The dichloromethane extract has exhibited better chromatogram in GC-MS analysis. All the solvents used were chromatographic grade purity.

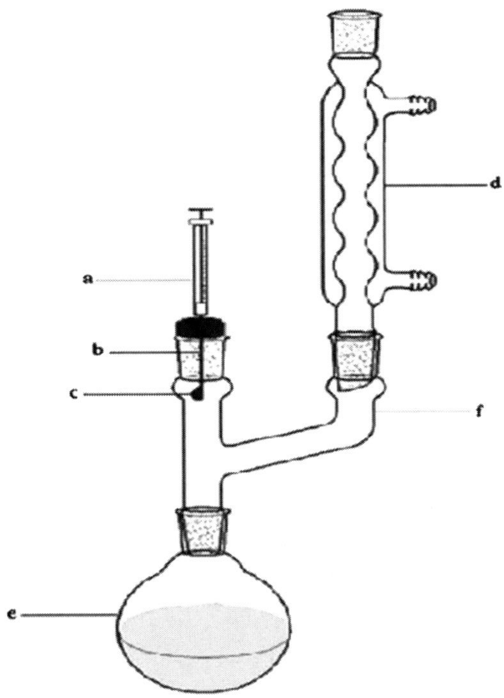

Figure 1. HD-SPME apparatus: (a) syringe (b) needle (c) microdrop (d) condenser (e) round bottom flask (f) claisen distillation head.

GC-MS Analysis

All extracts were analyzed on a GC-MS system which included a Shimadzu 2010 series of GC equipped with a AOC-20S automatic liquid sampler and interfaced directly to a QP2010 mass selective detector controlled via the accompanying data system. A 30-m DB-5MS capillary column (0.25 mm i.d., 0.25 µm film) was used. The temperature program used was as follows: initial temperature of 40 °C maintained for 1 min, then heated to 250°C at 10 °C/min, and subsequently to 300°C at 25°C/min, where it was held for 5 min. Injection volume was 1 µl in split-less mode. Helium was used as a carrier gas with 1 ml/min flow rate. Temperature of the injector was maintained at 260°C. A solvent delay of 5 min was maintained. Tuning was performed using the auto-tune feature with perfluorotributylamine; the electron multiplier voltage was nominally kept at 1,500 V. All data were obtained by collecting the full-scan mass spectra within the scan range of 40–550 amu.

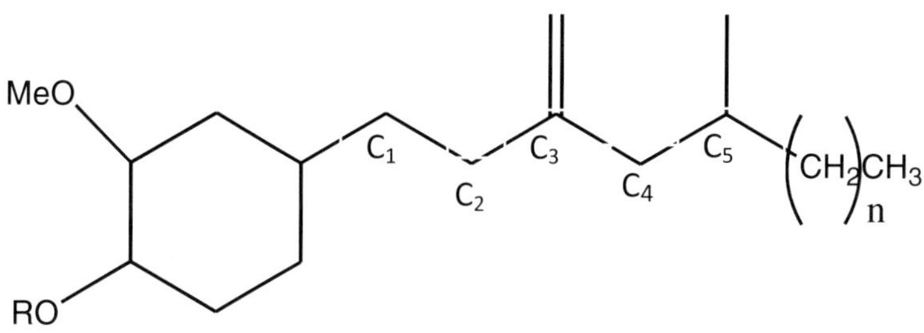

[6]- Gingerol ; n = 4; R = H ; M = 294

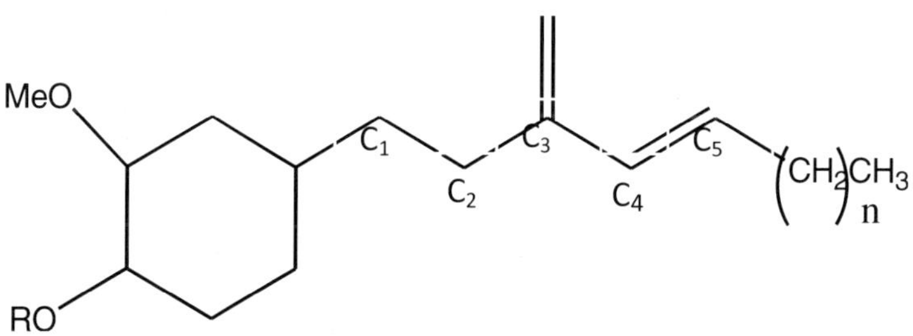

[8]- Shogaol ; n = 6; R = H ; M = 304

[10]- Shogaol ; n = 8; R = H ; M = 332

Figure 2. (Continued).

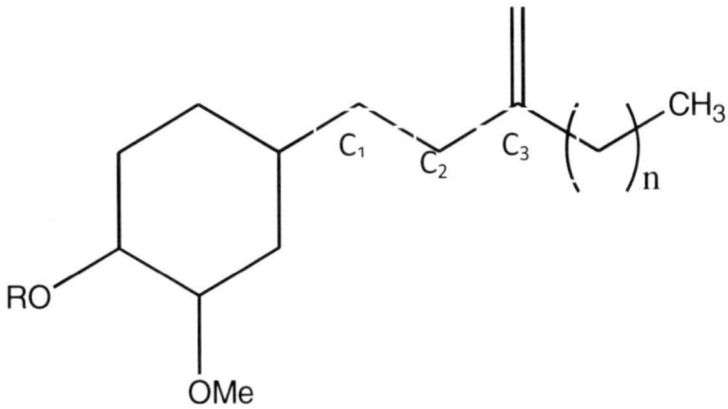

[6]- Paradol ; n = 6; R = H ; M = 278
[7]- Paradol ; n = 7; R = H ; M = 292

Figure 2. Some ginger pungent constituents.

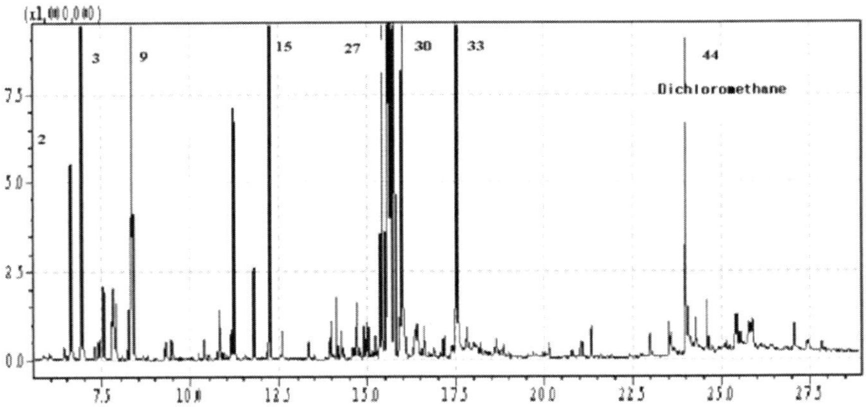

Figure 3. GC-MS total ion chromatogram of compounds in ginger using dichloromethane as a solvent.

RESULTS AND DISCUSSION

Non-polar compounds in ginger tissues were extracted with dichloromethane and thereafter analyzed by GC-MS. The electron impact ionization mass spectra obtained are reproducible and suitable for library matching, mass spectral collections being readily available. The compounds were identified using the Wiley 6.0 (Wiley, New York, NY, USA) and NIST mass spectral library Version 2.0 (NIST/ EPA/NIH, USA) and also by mass fragmentation pattern. Compound identifications indicated by the library search program as being >80% probable were viewed as being likely hits.

Some compounds present in small quantities in ginger tissues were not included in our analysis because they could not be readily identified due to insufficient mass spectrum quality or because of their relative concentrations that could not be adequately evaluated. About 49 compounds were identified; all the identified compounds could be broadly classified into four groups: monoterpenoids, sesquiterpenoids, gingerol-related compounds, and other compounds based on their chemical structures. The characteristic odor and flavor of ginger root is caused by a mixture of zingerone, shogaols, and gingerols, volatile oils that compose about 1% to 3% of the weight of fresh ginger.

The major compounds in the rhizome are α-zingiberene (25.55%), β-sesquiphellandrene (10.19%), β-phellandrene (9.08%), zingerone (8.04%), β-bisabolene (6.69%), α- farnesene (5.90%), camphene(5.09%), curcumene (4.03%), (E)-citral (3.70%), and [6]-gingerol (2.72%). Previous quantitative analyses of ginger (Govindarajan 1982) have shown that gingerols, a family of homologous compounds differentiated by the number of carbon atoms in their side chain, are the major pungent constituents, with [6]-gingerol [5-hydroxy-1-(40-hydroxy-30-methoxyphenyl) decan-3-one] being the most abundant. Another homologous series which also accounts for the pungency of ginger is the shogaol family, the dehydrated form of the gingerols, resulting from the elimination of the OH group at C-5 with the formation of a double bond between C-4 and C-5 (Figure 2). The presence of volatile oils, which were not investigated in this study, since we used dried ginger, makes the separation of minor volatile pungent components difficult.

The results of the quantitative analyses of [6]-gingerols and [8]- and [10]-shogaols in the CH_2Cl_2 extracts of ginger are summarized in Table 1. The most abundant in gingerols constituent was [6]-gingerol, representing nearly 2.72% followed by [8]- and [10]-shogaols at a meager level of 0.38% and 0.35%, respectively, suggests it could be from gingerols via dehydration or a naturally occurring minor constituent. For peak at m/z=137 was seen as the base peak, the most distinctive peak associated with the 4- hydroxy-3-methoxybenzyl cation ($C_8H_9O_2$) seen in the mass spectra of almost all gingerol (gingerols, shogaols, and paradols) compounds. Peaks with retention times RT <5 min were not studied because dichloromethane solvent elutes at 5 min (Figure 3). Compounds listed in Table 1 were detected in the region where RT >5 min. Other compounds in this region appeared to be mostly $C_{15}H_{22}$ and $C_{15}H_{24}$ sesquiterpenes and hydroxylated sesquiterpenes, gingerol isomers based on the observed molecular ion ([M]+) and fragmentation peaks (Yu et al. 1998; Sharma et al. 2002). A complicating factor in the present GC-MS analyses study was that some of the ginger compounds partially or completely thermally decomposed before they reached their retention time. Although some of these decomposition products may not be natural products, all are likely produced when ginger is used in cooking at high temperatures and subsequently eaten; this should increase interest in their presence in this study. Fortunately, only a few major types of thermal decomposition occur with ginger compounds. The gingerol comparisons show that [8]- and [10]-gingerols are almost completely decomposed before its RT and the zingerone (8.04%) are formed. In our case, we got more zingerone than gingerols indicating more gingerols are decomposed. The concentration of [8]- and [10]-shogaols in dry ginger is 0.73% signifies that while shogaols naturally co-occur with gingerols as minor constituents of ginger, here they may be derived largely from gingerols via dehydration.

Table 1. Relative percentage quantities of the compounds identified by GC-MS in the dried Korean ginger from the dichloromethane extract

Serial no.	Ginger constituents	Mol. formula	Mol. wt.	Area (%)
1	Tricyclene	$C_{10}H_{16}$	136	0.13
2	(1R)-(+)-α-Pinene	$C_{10}H_{16}$	136	2.13
3	Camphene	$C_{10}H_{16}$	136	5.09
4	4 (10)-Thujene	$C_{10}H_{16}$	136	0.11
5	α-Pinene	$C_{10}H_{16}$	136	0.16
6	β-Myrcene	$C_{10}H_{16}$	136	0.58
7	Octanal	$C_9H_{18}O$	142	0.72
8	α-Phellandrene	$C_{10}H_{16}$	136	0.49
9	β-Phellandrene	$C_{10}H_{16}$	136	9.08
10	(Z)-Alloocimene	$C_{10}H_{16}$	136	0.17
11	Linalool	$C_{10}H_{18}O$	154	0.12
12	Citronellal	$C_{10}H_{18}O$	154	0.13
13	(-)-Borneol	$C_{10}H_{18}O$	154	0.40
14	Neral	$C_{10}H_{16}O$	152	0.74
15	(E)-Citral	$C_{10}H_{16}O$	152	3.70
16	2-Undecanone	$C_{11}H_{22}O$	170	0.23
17	δ-Elemene	$C_{15}H_{24}$	204	0.13
18	α-Copaene	$C_{15}H_{24}$	204	0.29
19	β-Elemene	$C_{15}H_{24}$	204	0.56
20	(E)-α-Bergamotene	$C_{15}H_{24}$	204	0.20
21	Germacrene B	$C_{15}H_{24}$	204	0.49
22	(Z)-β-Farnesene	$C_{15}H_{24}$	204	0.27

Serial no.	Ginger constituents	Mol. formula	Mol. wt.	Area (%)
23	α-Caryophyllene	$C_{15}H_{24}$	204	0.30
24	Aromadendrene	$C_{15}H_{24}$	204	0.20
25	ar-Curcumene	$C_{15}H_{22}$	202	4.03
26	Germacrene D	$C_{15}H_{24}$	204	1.12
27	α-Zingiberene	$C_{15}H_{24}$	204	25.55
28	(E,E)- α-Farnesene	$C_{15}H_{24}$	204	5.90
29	β-Bisabolene	$C_{15}H_{24}$	204	6.69
30	β-Sesquiphellandrene	$C_{15}H_{24}$	204	10.19
31	β-elemene	$C_{15}H_{24}$	204	0.30
32	(E)-Nerolidol	$C_{15}H_{26}O$	222	0.36
33	Zingerone	$C_{11}H_{14}O_3$	194	8.04
34	Elemol	$C_{15}H_{26}O$	222	0.47
35	β-Eudesmol	$C_{15}H_{26}O$	222	0.10
36	Isoaromadendrene epoxide	$C_{15}H_{26}O$	222	0.10
37	(Z)-a-(E)-Bergamotol	$C_{15}H_{24}O$	220	0.08
38	Farnesal	$C_{15}H_{24}O$	220	0.10
39	trans-α-Bergamotene,	$C_{15}H_{24}$	204	0.10
40	(±)-(E)-Nuciferol	$C_{15}H_{22}O$	218	0.22
41	α-Longipinane	$C_{15}H_{24}$	204	0.24
42	Nerolidol	$C_{15}H_{26}O$	222	0.21
43	[6]-Paradol	$C_{17}H_{26}O_3$	278	0.19
44	[6]-Gingerol	$C_{17}H_{26}O_4$	294	2.72
45	[7]-Paradol	$C_{18}H_{28}O_3$	292	0.43
46	E-Retinal	$C_{20}H_{28}O$	284	0.45
47	[8]-Shogaol	$C_{19}H_{28}O_3$	304	0.38
48	[10]-Shogaol	$C_{21}H_{32}O_3$	332	0.35
49	α-Trans-sesquicyclogeraniol	$C_{15}H_{26}O$	222	0.10

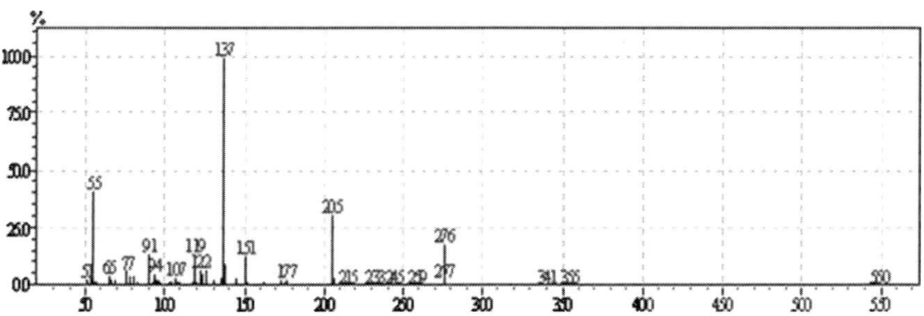

Figure 4. Mass spectrum compound44 ([6]-gingerol) listed in Table 1.

Compounds other than gingerols are identified using mass spectral library. However, the gingerols (gingerols, shogaols, and paradols) are identified by studying the mass spectrum fragmentation. Gingerol and paradol homologs were identified by comparison of their spectra with those of [6]-gingerol and [6]-paradol, respectively.

In the GC-MS spectra of [6]-gingerol (Figure 4), a notable feature was a peak at m/z=205, resulting from the cleavage of the C-5/C-6 bond in the dehydrated ions at m/z=276. Additional diagnostic peaks at m/z=177 (m/z=205-CO) and 151 (C- 2/C-3 cleavage) were seen as a minor fragmentation process.

The thermal degradation and dehydration ofcompounds, e.g., the [n]-gingerols, to aliphatic aldehydes and zingerones and to the corresponding [n]-shogaols under gas chromatographic conditions, thermal processing, and long-term storage has long been noted (Connell and Sutherland 1969; Connell and McLachian 1972; Mustafa et al. 1993).

The mass spectrum of gingerols are very similar to those of [6]- and [8]-shogaols except for the presence of a peak at m/z=194. The GC-MS spectrum of [8]-shogaol, reproduced in Figure 5, serves as a typical example. It is concluded from the above results that the higher members of gingerol homologs (n>8) because of their long retention times (even at temperatures as high as 300 °C), undergo complete thermal dehydration while the lower members suffer partial dehydration and isomerization as well.

Paradols are 5-deoxygingerols. The GC-MS spectrum of [6]-paradol, reproduced in Figure 6, shows a typical paradol fragmentation pattern. A base peak at m/z= 137, a C-3/C-4 fission peak at m/z=179.

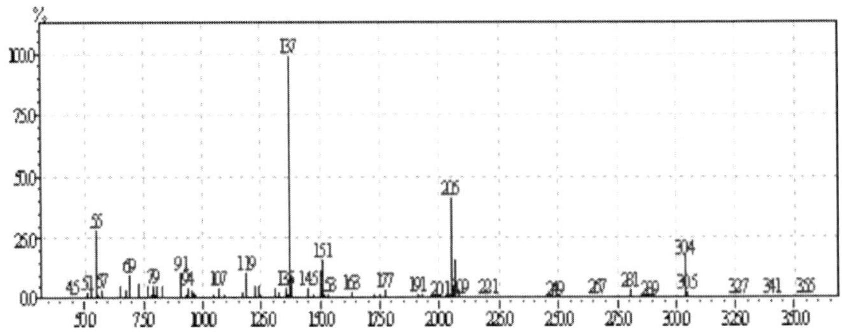

Figure 5. Mass spectrum of compound 47 ([8]-shogaol) listed in, Table 1.

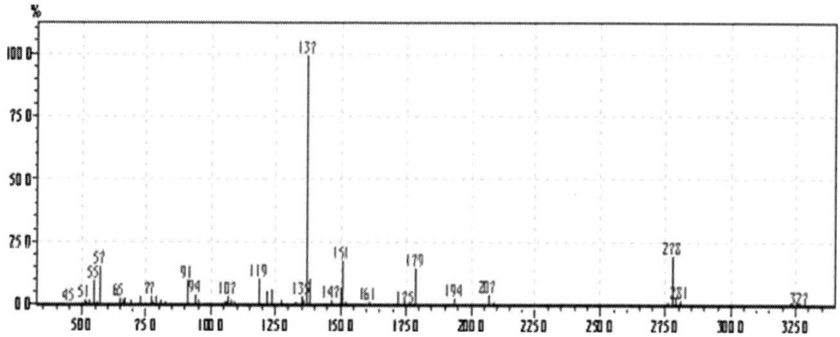

Figure 6. Mass spectrum of compound 43 ([6]-paradol) listed in Table 1.

CONCLUSION

In this paper, a relatively new method involving concurrent headspace solvent microextraction coupled with continuous hydrodistillation (HD-HSME) for analysis of the essential oil of ginger is reported. GC-MS method was developed and 49 compounds are identified. Some of the ginger compounds partially or completely were thermally decomposed. Some of these decomposition products likely produced when ginger is used in cooking at high temperatures and subsequently eaten; this should increase interest in the present study. The method has advantageous due to its shorter analysis time, minimal sample preparation and it can also be used in the quality standardization of ginger extracts for pharmaceutical production. The method also will be very useful for rapid screening purpose of plant samples for finding of high quality ginger under the plant breeding program and export quality of ginger species.

ACKNOWLEDGMENTS

One of the authors (D.C.B.) acknowledges the financial support from Brain Korea-21 Research Program. We thank Mrs. Bang Seon Ko for the assistance in operating GC-MS.

REFERENCES

Clark J, Dewan R, Locksley HD, Maynard R (1977). *J Chromatogr* 134:315.

Connell D, Sutherland MD (1969). *Aust J Chem* 22:1033.

Connell DW, McLachian R (1972). *J Chromatogr* 67(1):29.

Govindarajan VS (1982). *CRC Crit Rev Food Sci Nutr Part1* 17:1–96.

Harvey DJ (1981). *J Chromatogr* 212:75.

Kikuzaki H, Kawasaki Y, Nakatani N (1994). *ACS Symposium* Series 547.

Kiuchi F, Iwakami S, Shibuya M, Hanaoka F, Sankawa U (1992) *Chem Pharm Bull* 40:387.

Masada Y, Inoue T, Hashimoto K, Fuzioka M, Shiraki K (1973).

Masada Y, Inoue T, Hashimoto K, Fuzioka M, Uchino C (1974).

Mustafa T, Srivastava KC, Jensen KB (1993). *J Drug Dev* 6:25.

Park KK, Chun KS, Lee JM, Lee SS, Surh YJ (1998). *Cancer Lett* 129:139–144.

Sankawa U (1987). *The J. Traditional Sino-Japanese Medicine* 8(1):57.

Sharma RK, Sarma TC, Leclercq PA (2002). *J Essential Oilbearing Plants* 5:71.

Sivarajan VV, Balachandran I (1994). Calcutta: Oxford & IBH Publishing Co. Pvt. Ltd.

Srivasta KC (1986) Prostaglandins. *Leuko Med* 25:187.

Tanabe M, Chen YD, Saito K, Kano Y (1993). *Chem Pharm Bull* 41:710.

Yakugaku Zasshi. *J Pharm Soc Jap* 93(3):318.

Yakugaku Zasshi. *J Pharm Soc Jap* 94(6):735.

Yamahara J, Hatakeyama S, Taniguchi K, Kawamura M, Yoshikawa M (1992). *Yakugaku Zasshi* 112:645.

Yamahara J, Huang Q, Li Y, Xu L, Fujimura H (1990). *Chem PharmBull* 38(2):430.

Yamahara J, Mochizwki M, Huang QR, Matsuda H, Fujimura H(1988). *J Ethnopharmacol* 23:299.

Yoshikawa M, Yamaguchi S, Kunimi K, Matsuda H, Okuno Y, Yamahara J, Murakami N (1994). *Chem Pharm Bull* 42:1226.

Yu Z, Wu H, Ding J (1998). *Yunnan Zhiwu Yanjiu* 20:113.

In: Ginger
Editor: Janine L. Perry
ISBN: 978-1-63482-020-2

Chapter 7

THE ANTIMICROBIAL ACTIVITY OF SOME MEDICINAL PLANTS AGAINST MULTIDRUG RESISTANCE BACTERIA WHICH CAUSES MASTITIS

Shaza Anwar Al Laham[1]*
and Frdoos Mohammad Al Fadel[2]
Department of Pharmacology and Toxicology, Faculty of Pharmacy,
Damascus University, Damascus, Syria

Researchers have for many decades been trying to develop new broad-spectrum antibiotics against the infectious diseases caused by bacteria. Prolonged usage of these broad-spectrum antibiotics has led to the emergence of drug resistance. Resistance to antimicrobial agents has become an increasingly important and pressing global problem. There is a tremendous need for novel antimicrobial agents from different sources.

Plants used in traditional medicine are still understudied, particularly in clinical microbiology. So seeking for the *in vitro* antimicrobial activity of natural compounds such as polyphenols from ethnomedicinal plants on pathogenic bacteria is a new challenge.

Therefore, we investigated the possibility of the plants having the capacity to confront these bacteria.

* Corresponding author: Shaza Anwar Al Laham. Department of Pharmacology and Toxicology, Faculty of Pharmacy, Damascus University, Damascus, Syria. Tel: +96-30113136591. E-mail: Lahamshaza@gmail.com. mobile: 0963933375655. Fax: 0963-011-3312041.

SCREENING THE ANTIMICROBIAL ACTIVITY OF SOME MEDICINAL PLANTS AGAINST MULTIDRUG RESISTANT *ESCHERICHIA COLI TYPE (1)*

ABSTRACT

The increasing number of *Escherichia coli* causing mastitis and of bacteria resistant to conventional antibiotics has become a serious problem in recent years. So the search for new antibiotics and alternative products to solve this problem is the question of the age.

The Aim: This research aims to investigate the effect of the extracts prepared from different parts of the following plants: *Olea europea Linn (Oleaceae)* ، *Myrtus communis Linn (Liliaceae)*، *Majorana syriacus Linn (Laminaceae)*، *Zingiber officinale Linn (Zingiberaceae)*، *Achillea falcata Linn (Asteraceae)* against resistant *Escherichia coli Type (1).*

Material and Methods: Investigation began for *E.coli* bacteria in 667 milk samples. The bacteria were identified culturally, morphologically and biochemically. Antibiotic susceptibility testing against *E.coli* by Kirby-Bauer disk diffusion method was conducted. Then using the blood agar, MacConkey agar, salmonella - shigella agar, and biochemical testing method [API 20 E testing Enterobacteriaceae] were made to type *E.coli*. Plants were extracted with water, absolute alcohol, then ether using a soxhlet apparatus and rotary vacuum evaporator. Then extracts susceptibility testing against antibiotic resistant *E.coli Type (1)* were studied.

Results: E. coli was defined as oxidase negative, indole positive, catalase positive. The studied antibiotics did not show any antibacterial effect against *E.coli*. By the results of the biochemical analysis (API20e) on resistant *E.coli*, *E.coli type (1)* was 33.35% of the total number of samples. The anti-bacterial effect against *E.coli type (1)* of ethanol extracts prepared from different parts of the studied plants were variant, whereas the *Myrtus communis* extract effectively has the most powerful antibacterial effect for these bacteria, while the *Zingiber officinale* extract has the lowest influence.

Conclusion: the ethanol extracts of studied plants had the anti-bacterial effect against resistant *E.coli type (1)*, which causes mastitis.

Keywords: Olea europea, Myrtus communis, Achillea falcate, Majorana syriacus, Zingiber officinale ,E.coli, resistant bacteria

INTRODUCTION

Mastitis is the inflammation of the milk gland with physical, chemical and microbiological changes characterized by an increase in somatic cells especially, leukocytes in the milk. This disease possesses the risk of transmitting zoonotic diseases like *tuberculosis, brucellosis, leptospirosis* and *streptococcal* sore throat to humans [1]. The inflammation of the mammary gland is usually a consequence of invasion and colonization in the secretory tissue by one or more microorganisms, especially *Staphylococcus aureus, Streptococcus agalactiae, Streptococcus dysgalactiae, Streptococcus uberis*, and *Escherichia coli* [2]. *Escherichia coli* are facultative anaerobes in the normal intestinal flora of humans and animals; however, pathogenic strains of these bacteria are an important cause of bacterial infections. In humans, these strains are the foremost cause of urinary tract infections. Infection with Shiga toxin–producing E. coli (STEC) may also cause complications including thrombocytopenic purpura, severe hemorrhagic colitis, and hemolytic uremic syndrome [3]. Multi-drug resistant strains of *Escherichia coli* are widely distributed. Thus, it is an urgent need to find out new antimicrobial agents. For this reason, researchers are increasingly turning their attention to herbal products, looking for new ways to develop better drugs against multidrug resistant microbe strains. Philip et al. reveled that none of the extracts of *Pereskia bleo, pereskia grandifoila, Curcuma aeruginosa Roxb., Curcuma zedoria, curcuma mangga, curcuma inodora aff.Blatter, and zingiber officinale var.* that used by Malaysia traditional health care systems, showed activity against *Escherichia coli* [4].

Myrtus communis Linn back to the Myrtaceae, is an evergreen herb, grows throughout the Mediterranean area and has been used for medicine, food and spice since ancient times. In folk medicine, the fruit of the plant is used in the treatment of various infectious diseases, including diarrhea and dysentery, whereas the leaves are used as antiseptic and anti-inflammatory agents, as well as in the therapy of urinary diseases. The leaves contain tannins, flavonoids such as quercetin, catechin and myricetin derivatives and volatile oils [5]. Many studies have shown its antibacterial effect [6, 7]. ***Achillea falcata Linn*** backs to the *Asteraceae*, is an herb perennial. The flowers have yellow color, which grows in the Badia region of Syria. Indigenous uses of ***Achillea*** species are diuretic, emmenagogic agents, wound healing, curing stomachache, diarrhea and antispasmodic, and are used in cosmetics. Recent studies reported that *Achillea* species had constituents such as flavonoids (aglycones & glycosides), sesquiterpene lactones and essential oils, the major constituent are 1,8-cineole, camphor, piperitone and ascaridole [8]. Some studies have pointed its anti-bacterial effect [9]. The ***Olea europea*** Linn from the *Oleaceae*, is an evergreen long-lasting fruit tree, and is rooted in the Mediterranean region [9]. Olive leaves are a good source of several antioxidants including oleuropeoside compounds such as oleuropein and verbascoside, and flavonoid compounds such as luteolin, luteolin-7-glucoside, apigenin-7-glucoside, diosmetin, diosmetin-7-glucoside, rutin and catechin, and simple phenolic compounds such as tyrosol, hydroxytyrosol, vanillin, vanillic acid and caffeic acid [10]. Most of these phenolic compounds have shown to possess substantial antimicrobial and antioxidant activities *in vitro*, while other non-phenolic components such as aldehydes have also been studied for their antimicrobial properties [5]. A number of studies revealed the antibacterial, antiviral, and antifungal compounds [10, 11]. *Zingiber officinale Linn (Zingiberaceae),* is a minor chemical irritant, and has a sialagogue action. Mature *Zingiber officinale (Ginger)* roots are fibrous and nearly dry. Its roots are used as spice in cooking [12]. *Ginger* possesses other interesting pharmacological and physiological properties. For instance, it acts as an anti-inflammatory, analgesic, antipyretic, anti-hepatotoxic and cardiotonic substance. Several studies also revealed its anti-bacterial effect [13, 14]. The main constituents of Ginger are sesquiterpenoids with zingiberene as the main component. Gingerone, shoagoles and gingerols, volatile oils [12]. Gingerol-related components have been reported to possess antimicrobial and antifungal properties, as well as several pharmaceutical properties [15].

Finally *Majorana syriacus Linn (Marjoram or Origanum syriaca L.)* (Laminaceae family). The genus Origanum majorana L. is an aromatic, perennial, herbaceous plant. The plant has been used as a flavouring and herbal spice from time immemorial. The plant is pungent, bitter, hot, stomachic, anthelmintic, alexipharmic, useful in diseases of the heart and blood, fevers, leucoderma and inflammation. The plant is reported to possess antibacterial activity [16].

The major volatiles and semi-volatiles of Palestinian wild M. syriaca are, a-phellandrene, a-pinene, b-myrecene, o-cymene, p-cymene, c-terpinene, thymol, and carvacrol [17]. Marjoram (Origanum majorana),is widely used in cooking, marjoram has a long history of medicinal use, by the Greeks as an antidote to poisoning and snake venom, by the Romans for stomach disorders and more recently for digestive, antispasmodic and sedative properties [18].

Material and Methods

1. Preparing Plant Extracts

Myrtus communis, Olea europea, and *Majorana syriacus* leaves, and *Achillea falcata* flowers, were collected in the early morning hours during the period from June to August from Damascus rural area, while the Zingiber officinale roots were purchased from Damascus markets, which were identified by Prof. Dr. Anwar Al-Khatib from Damauscs University. Plant parts were extracted separately by continuous extraction device (Soxhlet apparatus), adopted method described by Wang [19] for preparing plant extracts by organic solvents, which are respectively: water, absolute ethanol, and then Light Petroleum.

2. Sampling Method

667 milk samples were collected from dairy cows with clinical mastitis (as veterinary diagnosis). These samples were investigated for the presence of *Escherichia coli*. The bacteria were identified culturally, morphologically and biochemically. Microscopic examination was conducted after 24 hours of incubation on blood agar (HiMedia) plates. All of the following tests were conducted: oxidase, catalase, Indole test.

3. A Bacterial Growth Inhibition Test of Antibiotics by the Disk Diffusion Method

Pure cultures of udder pathogens were tested for antibacterial susceptibility by the disc diffusion method (Kirby-Bauer Disk Diffusion Susceptibility Test Protocol) using the 15 antimicrobial substances (Becton Dikinson, Microbiology Systems, MD, USA)on Mueller- Hinton agar medium. Testing was performed according to the recommendation of the Clinical and Laboratory Standards Institute (CLSI) document M100-S17 in 2009 [20, 21].

5 mm diameter standard discs contain certain concentrations of the following antibiotics (Bioanalyse): amikacin (30 μg), Cephalexin (30 μg), cephalothin(30 μg), Doxycyclin(30 μg), Cefadroxil (30 μg), ciprofloxacin (5

μg), chloramphenicol (30 μg), gentamicin (10 μg), Norfloxacin (10 μg), Oxytetracycline (30 μg), Pefloxacin (5 μg), Oxacillin (1 μg), Enrofloxacin (5 μg), tetracycline (30 μg), and Amoxicillin (25 μg). The resistance breakpoints were those defined by the National Committee for Clinical Laboratory Standards (NCCLS, 2000) for gram-positive bacteria [20, 21] .Negative controls were prepared using the same solvents as used to prepare the extracts. The size of the zones of inhibition was measured.

4. Analytical Profile Index Technique (API20e)

The bacterial colonies, which were susceptibil to the antibiotic, were abandoned.

23 differential biochemical tests were performed by API20E system (Analytical Profile Index) manufactured by Bio Merieux, France:

a) Investigate the effect of enzymes: 2 - nitrophenyl-βD-galacto-pyranoside, Arginine dihydrolase, oxidase.
b) Decarboxylation Interactions of amino acids: L-lysine, L-omithine.
c) Deaminase interaction of the amino acid: L-tryptophan.
d) Fermentation reactions of the following sugars: D-glucose, D-mannitol, Inositol, D-sorbitol, L-rhamnose, D-sucrose, D-melibiose, Amygdaline Arabinose.
e) Production reactions: indole, Asitoen.
f) Reactions produce gases: hydrogen sulphide, nitrogen, nitrogen oxide.
g) Study the interactions of Recipes: gelatin diluted, citrate use, hydrolysis of urea (urease).

Then for stereotyping resistance *E. coli,* the selective media according to the method of [22], were McCoonky agar, XLD agar, Salmonella – shigella agar.

5. A Bacterial Growth Inhibition Test of Plant Extracts by the Disk Diffusion Method against *E. Coli* Type (1) that Showed Resistance to All Antibiotics

Bacterial suspension was emulsified with Agar-agar medium to test the susceptibility of plant extracts. Sterile filter paper discs (5 mm) were soaked with 5mcl of the diluted extracts (66 mg/ml) of pericarp, leaves, flowers ,seeds in ethanol, water ,and petroleum ether, so that each disc was impregnated with 0.33 mg / tablet. Control disks also prepared with absolute ethanol, Water, and petroleum ether. Results were expressed as the percentage of inhibition of bacterial growth, determined by comparing it with Control disks, and standard susceptibility disks [23].

RESULTS

1. Identification of the Bacteria

Bacteria samples that gave us the following results were selected:

Staining with a gram stain: Gram-negative, non-motile, straight rods with round edges, no capsule, and non sporing bacteria that form compatible with reference [22, 24].

2. The Results of Biochemical Tests

Biochemical confirmation of the strains was performed and *E. coli* was defined as oxidase negative, indole positive, catalase positive. These results depended on Al-Rifai study [24].

3. Antimicrobial Susceptibility Results against *E. Coli*

Bacterial colonies showed resistant to all studied antibiotics, based on the criteria of NCCLS2000 [25], and to the standard's leaflet of antibiotic discs from the manufacturer. These colonies were selected to test the plant extracts.

Table 1. The percentage of antimicrobial sensibility to *E. coli*

Antibiotics	diameters zones of inhibition (mm)	Antimicrobial susceptibility results	Percentage of sensitive bacteria %
Oxytetracycline (T)	9,2±1,09	resistant	98,89
Amoxicillin(AX)	8,4±0,8	resistant	91,59
Oxacillin(OX)	7,6±0.9	resistant	88,75
Cefadroxil(CER)	7,2±0,8	resistant	93,14

Table 1. (Continued)

Antibiotics	diameters zones of inhibition (mm)	Antimicrobial susceptibility results	Percentage of sensitive bacteria %
Pefloxacin(PEF)	9,2±1,1	resistant	94,09
Amikacin(AK)	8±1,2	resistant	96,92
Tetracyclin(TE)	7,9±0,7	resistant	90,11
Ciprofloxacin(CIP)	9,3±0,8	resistant	87,49
Norfloxacin(NOR)	6,9±1,4	resistant	84.04
Gentamycin(CN)	8,5±1,3	resistant	78,62
Chloramphenicol(C)	8,7±0,9	resistant	95,76
Enrofloxacin(ENR)	10,9±0,5	resistant	79,57
Doxycyclin(DO)	8,5±1,2	resistant	87,18
Cephalexin(CL)	7,4±0,8	resistant	90.64
Cephalotin(KF)	9,7±1,3	resistant	93.51

4. The Results of Analytical Profile Index Technique (API20e)

According to the data contained in the annex with these tests the results of these tests were depended. The results of the biochemical analysis (API20e) after the end of the incubation period, according to the method used in the directory of the test facilities, were: 5144512 as a result of this reading on *E.coli type (1)*.

Table 2. Shows the results of (API20E) technique

Test	**Test result**
Urea	-
Tryptophan deaminase	-
Indol	+
Voges-proskauer eactin	-
Gelatinase	-
Glucose	+
Mannitol	+
Inositol	-

Test	Test result
Sorbitol	+
Ramnose	+
Saccarose	-
Melibiose	-
Amygdalin	-
Arabinose	+
Oxidase	

So as a result 223(33.43%) out of total number 667 samples were gotten of *E. coli type (1)*.

5. Colonial and Cultural Characters

These results were depended according to [22, 24].

- Growth on blood agar: circular colonies, white, and smooth with a fecal odor.
- Growth on McCoonky agar: the growth of red colonies.
- Growth on XLD agar (xylose lysine desoxycholate agar) European pharmacopoeia: yellow colonies with wet strength, and with zone of yellow precipitation around the colonies.
- Growth on Salmonella – shigella agar: red colonies.

6. The Results of Antibacterial Efficacy of Plant Extracts against *E. Coli* Type (1)

The petroleum ether, and water extract from studied plants were not active against *E. coli type I (1)* (diameters of zone of inhibition were zero).

As shown in Table (3), the ethanol extracts of various plants showed antibacterial activity against *E. coli type(1)*, with the diameters of zone of inhibition ranging between 6 and 20 mm.

Mean inhibition zones indicate that *Myrtus communis leaves* extracts exert a powerful effect on *E.coli type(1),* while the Zingiber officinale extract has the lowest influence.

Table 3. Antibacterial activity of different extracts of studied plants

Plant	Inhibition zones of plant extracts (mm) mean ±S.D	Percentage of sensitive bacteria %
Control/5 μm	0	0
Myrtus communis leaves	20±1,3	90.4
Achillea falcata flowers	18±0,7	84.35
Olea Europea leaves	16±1,2	68.55
Majorana syriacus leaves	8±1,08	74.55
Zingiber officinale roots	6±1,1	45.36

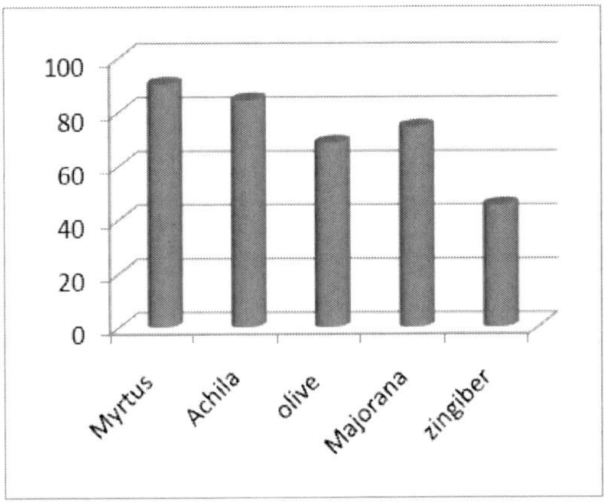

Figure 1. Percentage of sensitive bacteria.

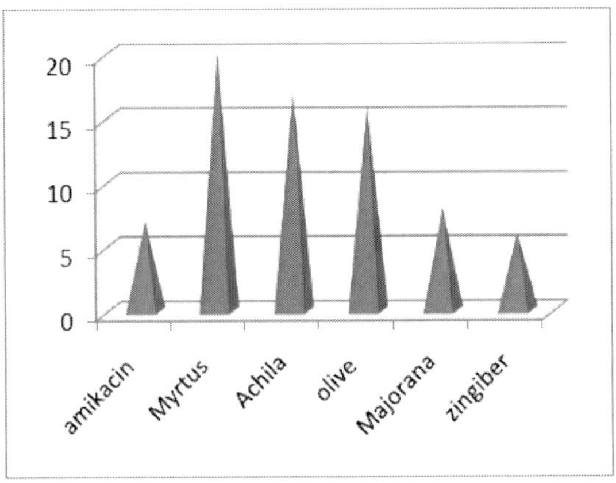

Figure 2. Mean of inhibition diameter of plants extract and Amikacin against *E. coli type (1)*.

DISCUSSION

In the present study, antibacterial activity in the leaf extracts of various plants against multidrug resistant pathogenic bacteria *Escherichia coli type* (1) was evaluated by vitro agar disc diffusion method, *E.coli* was resistant to all antimicrobials assayed, where the ethanol extract exhibits maximum antibacterial activity against *Escherichia coli* type (1). The present study demonstrates that ethanol extract, not aqucous, or ether petroleum extracts, exhibits an inhibitory effect on *E.coli* type (1) growth. This may in part be due to different chemical compositions between aqueous and ethanol extracts.

The results showed variation in the antimicrobial properties of plant extracts (Table 3). The ethanol extracts showed strong activity (inhibition zone 20-16 mm), and weak inhibition (zone 8-6 mm).

As a result ,the plants were arranged according to their effect against *E.coli type(1)* to find that the major effect was achieved by the ethanol extracts from *Myrtus communis* leaves, followed by *Achillea falcata* flowers, and *Olea Europea* leaves extract. While the *Majorana syriacus,* and Zingiber officinale leaves has the weakest's influence. Considering the large number of different groups of chemical compounds present in plants, it is most likely that their antibacterial activity is not attributed to one specific mechanism but that there are several targets in the cell. The antimicrobial potency of plants is believed to be due to, saponins, phenolic compounds, essential oils and flavonoids [26]. Most of the studies on the mechanism of phenolic compounds have focused on their effects on cellular membranes. They have been seen to attack not only cell walls and cell membranes, thereby affecting their permeability and the release of intracellular constituents, but also to interfere with membrane functions such as electron transport, enzyme activity or nutrient uptake. Thus, active phenolic compounds might have several targets which could lead to the inhibition of bacteria [27]. As in khder article these compounds were found in denature proteins and block enzymes and subsequently the bacteria losses its activity [6]. *Myrtus communis* leaves contain different polyphenol classes as flavonols and galloyl derivatives, their antimicrobial mode of action was related to the presence of phenolic compounds [27]. More over *Myrtucomlone A&B* are considered as two new acylphloraglucinols identified in the leaves and fruits of *M.communis* and have shown a significant antimicrobial effect against bacteria. The inhibition effect may be regarded to present Tannin via producing hydrogen bonds with proteins, which convert its structure and lead to block the protein synthesis, and tannins is considered as a phenolic compounds of plants [6]. So the inhibition effect of *Myrtus communis* towards

E.coli type(1) isolates may refer to the polyphenolic and Tannin they contain. Information about the antimicrobial activity of *Achillea* extracts is limited. The study of the 13 Turkish *Achillea* species showed that not all of the *Achillea* species possess antibacterial activity. *Achillea falcata* showed mild to low antibacterial activity [9]. Also water-insoluble parts of the methanolic extracts exhibited slight or no activity [28]. In contrast at Stojanović's study, extracts of several species of *Achillea* possess a broad spectrum of antimicrobial activity against tested strains *Staphylococcus aureus*, and *Escherichia coli* [29, 30], which matched our results. The composition of the extract of *Achillea clavennae* are alkanes, fatty acids, monoterpenes, guaiane sesquiterpenes, and flavonoids (apigenin and centaureidin) [29]. The genus *Achillea* has been extensively studied in regard to its flavonoids and sesquiterpene lactones. Flavonoids possess antimicrobial properties and several investigations have examined the relationship between flavonoid structure and antibacterial activity. Promising evidence has clearly shown that sesquiterpene lactones derived from several different plant species have significant antimicrobial activity in vitro [9]. Researchers have published numerous studies concluding that *olive* leafs active ingredient, oleuropein and its derivative hydroxytyrosol act as a natural antibiotic agent. Oleuropein has been shown to have strong antimicrobial activity against both Gram-negative and Gram-positive bacteria, as well as mycoplasma. Oleuropein and other phenolic compounds completely inhibit the development of *Klebsiella pneumoniae, Escherichia coli* and *B.* cereus [31]. Phenolic structures similar to oleuropein seem to produce its antibacterial effect by damaging the bacterial membrane and/or disrupting cell peptidoglycans [32]. However, the exact mechanism of the antimicrobial effect of oleuropein is still not completely confirmed, although some authors have suggested that it is due to the presence of the ortho-diphenolic system (catechol) [31]. Other researchers concluded that oleuropeins can enhance nitric oxide production in mouse macrophages. By increasing nitric oxide production, oleuropein appears to arm the macrophages against endotoxins. Interestingly, oleuropein only increase nitric oxide production when endotoxins were present [33]. Ethanol extract of *Ginger* inhibited *E.coli* showing 9 mm diameter [34], as our study. *Ginger* extract found to have moderate antibacterial properties against *E. coli* serogroups O8 and O88, while it did not show any antibacterial activity against all other serogroups of *E. coli* [35]. In contrast, Sofia at el. reported that the *Ginger* extract showed negligible antibacterial activity against *Escherichia coli, staphylococcus aureus* and *Bacillus cereus* [36], and no effect not even by hexane, ethyl acetate, water, and methanol extracts [13]. Also aqueous extracts of *Zingiber officinale* did not exhibit *in vitro* any inhibition on the growth of *E. coli* [37], which confirmed the result of our study. The methanol extract of *Origanum majorana* against the *E.coli* has 18 mm diameter Zone of inhibition [16], while our study showed 8 mm. The methanol extract of shade dried aerial parts of *O.majorana* had showed variable activity against *Bacillus subtilis,B. megaterium, Escherichia coli, Proteus vulgaris, Pseudomonas aeruginosa* and *Staphylococcus aureus* [16]. The antibacterial activity exhibited by *Origanum majorana* essential oil, and The n-hexane extract of Four sweet marjoram *(Origanum majorana)* fractions have been demonstrated [38]. In contrast, at Joshi's study the most resistant bacteria to *Origanum majorana* extract were *E.coli* [39].

We believe that this is the first study on the antibacterial effect of Achillea, and majorana on this type of bacteria, Escherichia coli type (1).

CONCLUSION

The ethanol extracts of *Myrtus communis, Achillea falcata, Olea Europea, Majorana syriacus,* and Zingiber officinale showed variant antibacterial activity against resistant *Escherichia coli Type (1),* which causes mastitis. *Myrtus, Achillea,* and *olive* had beaten out all the strongest antibiotics in possession the antibacterial effect on these bacteria.

REFERENCES

[1] Bachaya, H; Iqbal, Z; Muhammad, G; Yousaf, A; Ali, H. Subclinical mastitis in buffaloes in Attock district of Punjab (Pakistan). *Pakistan Veterinary Journal.* 2005;25(3):134.

[2] Martín, BS; Kruze, J; Morales, MA; Agüero, H; Iragüen ,D; Espinoza, S; et al. Antimicrobial Resistance in Bacteria Isolated From Dairy Herds in Chile. *The International Journal of Applied Research in Veterinary Medicine.* 2009;4(7).

[3] Schroeder, CM; Meng, J; Zhao, S; DebRoy, C; Torcolini, J; Zhao, C; et al. Antimicrobial resistance of Escherichia coli O26, O103, O111, O128, and O145 from animals and humans. Emerging Infectious Diseases. 2002;8(12):1409.

[4] Brazier, J; Levett, P; Stannard, A; Phillips, K; Willis, A. Antibiotic susceptibility of clinical isolates of clostridia. *Journal of antimicrobial chemotherapy*. 1985;15(2):181-5.

[5] Naziri, Z; Rajaian, H; Firouzi, R. Antibacterial effects of Iranian native sour and sweet pomegranate (Punica granatum) peel extracts against various pathogenic bacteria. *Iranian Journal of Veterinary Research*. 2012;13(4):282-8.

[6] Khder, AK. Effect of Allium sativum and Myrtus communis on the elimination of antibiotic resistance and swarming of Proteus mirabilis. *Jordan Journal of Biological Sciences (JJBS)*. 2008:3124.

[7] Al-Anbori, DK; Al-Nimer, MS; Al-Weheb, AM. Athraa M:Antibacterial activity of ethanolic extract of Myrtus communis. L leaves against salivary Mutans streptococci. *Saudi Dental Journal*. 2008;20(3):82-7.

[8] Katzung, BG; Masters, SB; Trevor, AJ. Basic & clinical pharmacology: Lange Medical Books/McGraw-Hill Toronto; 2001.

[9] Karaalp, C; Yurtman, AN; Karabay; Yavasoglu, NU. Evaluation of antimicrobial properties of Achillea L. flower head extracts. *Pharmaceutical biology*. 2009;47(1):86-91.

[10] Pereira, AP; Ferreira, IC; Marcelino, F; Valentão, P; Andrade, PB; Seabra, R; et al. Phenolic compounds and antimicrobial activity of olive (Olea europaea L. Cv. Cobrançosa) leaves. *Molecules*. 2007;12(5):1153-62.

[11] Bisignano, G; Tomaino, A; Cascio, RL; Crisafi, G; Uccella, N; Saija, A. On the in-vitro antimicrobial activity of oleuropein and hydroxytyrosol. *Journal of pharmacy and pharmacology*. 1999;51(8):971-4.

[12] Marks, SL; Kather, EJ. Antimicrobial susceptibilities of canine Clostridium difficile and Clostridium perfringens isolates to commonly utilized antimicrobial drugs. *Veterinary microbiology*. 2003;94(1):39-45.

[13] Philip, K; Malek, SNA; Sani, W; Shin, SK; Kumar, S; Lai, HS; et al. Antimicrobial activity of some medicinal plants from Malaysia. *American Journal of Applied Sciences*. 2009;6(8):1613-7.

[14] Akoachere, J; Ndip, R; Chenwi, E; Ndip, L; Njock, T; Anong, D. Antibacterial effects of Zingiber Officinale and Garcinia Kola on respiratory tract pathogens. *East African medical journal*. 2006;79(11):588-92.

[15] Park, M; Bae, J; Lee, DS. Antibacterial activity of [10]-gingerol and [12]-gingerol isolated from ginger rhizome against periodontal bacteria. *Phytotherapy Research*. 2008;22(11):1446-9.

[16] Leeja, L; Thoppil, J. Antimicrobial activity of methanol extract of Origanum majorana L.(Sweet marjoram). *Journal of Environmental Biology*. 2007;28(1):145.
[17] Abu-Lafi, S; Odeh, I; Dewik, H; Qabajah, M; Hanuš, L; Dembitsky, V. Thymol and carvacrol production from leaves of wild Palestinian Majorana syriaca. *Bioresource technology*. 2008;99(9):3914-8.
[18] Evans, WC. Trease and Evans Pharmacognosy. 15th ed ed: WB Saunders company Ltd; 2002.
[19] Wang, L; Weller, CL. Recent advances in extraction of nutraceuticals from plants. *Trends in Food Science & Technology*. 2006;17(6):300-12.
[20] Hudzicki, J. Kirby-Bauer Disk Diffusion Susceptibility Test Protocol. Kirby-Bauer Disk Diffusion Susceptibility Test Protocol. 2009.
[21] Wilker, MA; Cockerill, FR; Craig, WA; Dudley, MN; Eliopoulos, GM; Hecht, DW. M100-S17 Performance Standards for Antimicrobial Susceptibility Testing;Seventeenth Informational Supplement. 2007; 27 (1).
[22] Ebeid M. microbiology. 4th ed: Publications of the University of Damascus; 2000.
[23] Pradeep, B;Manojbabu, M; Palaniswamy, M. Antibacterial Activity of Punica granatum L. Against Gastro Intestinal Tract Infection Causing Organisms. *Ethnobotanical Leaflets*. 2008;2008(1):143.
[24] Al-Rifai, I; Alomar, A. special Microbiology 2007:106-7.
[25] Standards NCfCL. NCCLS Antimicrobial Susceptibility Testing: National Committee for Clinical Laboratory Standards; 1992.
[26] Aboaba, O; Efuwape, B. Antibacterial properties of some Nigerian species. *Bio Res Comm*. 2001;13:183-8.
[27] Amensour, M; Bouhdid, S; Fernández-López, J; Idaomar, M; Senhaji, NS; Abrini, J. Antibacterial activity of extracts of Myrtus communis against food-borne pathogenic and spoilage bacteria. *International Journal of Food Properties*. 2010;13(6):1215-24.
[28] Candan, F; Unlu, M; Tepe, B; Daferera, D; Polissiou, M; Sökmen, A; et al. Antioxidant and antimicrobial activity of the essential oil and methanol extracts of Achillea millefolium subsp millefolium Afan.(Asteraceae). *Journal of Ethnopharmacology*. 2003;87(2):215-20.
[29] Stojanović, G; Radulović, N; Hashimoto, T; Palić, R. In vitro antimicrobial activity of extracts of four Achillea species: The composition of Achillea clavennae L.(Asteraceae) extract. *Journal of ethnopharmacology*. 2005;101(1):185-90.

[30] Tajik, H; Jalali, FSS; Sobhani, A; Shahbazi, Y; Zadeh, MS. In vitro assessment of antimicrobial efficacy of alcoholic extract of Achillea millefolium in comparison with penicillin derivatives. *Journal of Animal and Veterinary Advances*. 2008;7(4):508-11.

[31] Omar, SH. Oleuropein in olive and its pharmacological effects. *Scientia pharmaceutica*. 2010;78(2):133.

[32] Caturla, N; Pérez-Fons, L; Estepa, A; Micol, V. Differential effects of oleuropein, a biophenol from Olea europaea, on anionic and zwiterionic phospholipid model membranes. *Chemistry and physics of lipids*. 2005;137(1):2-17.

[33] Visioli, F; Bellosta, S; Galli, C. Oleuropein, the bitter principle of olives, enhances nitric oxide production by mouse macrophages. *Life sciences*. 1998;62(6):541-6.

[34] Hamad, M; Habra, N; Kalb-Allose, A. Isolated of Clostridium perfringens from intestinal bacteriotoxemia cases in the province of Hama. *Al-Baath University journal*. 2009;31(2).

[35] Indu, M; Hatha, A; Abirosh, C; Harsha, U; Vivekanandan, G. Antimicrobial activity of some of the south-Indian spices against serotypes of Escherichia coli, Salmonella, Listeria monocytogenes and Aeromonas hydrophila. *Brazilian Journal of Microbiology*. 2006;37(2):153-8.

[36] Alexander, CJ; Citron, DM; Brazier, JS; Goldstein, E. Identification and antimicrobial resistance patterns of clinical isolates of Clostridium clostridioforme, Clostridium innocuum, and Clostridium ramosum compared with those of clinical isolates of Clostridium perfringens. *Journal of clinical microbiology*. 1995;33(12):3209-15.

[37] Rahman, S; Parvez, AK; Islam, R; Khan, MH. Antibacterial activity of natural spices on multiple drug resistant Escherichia coli isolated from drinking water, Bangladesh. *Annals of clinical microbiology and antimicrobials*. 2011;10(1):10.

[38] Chomicz, L; Kazimierczuk, Z; Kozlowska, M; Laudy, A; Napiorkowski, A ; Starosciak, B. Antimicrobial and antiprotozoal effect of sweet marjoram (Origanum majorana L.). *Acta Scientiarum Polonorum*. 2010.

[39] Joshi, B; Lekhak, S; Sharma, A. Antibacterial Property of Different Medicinal Plants: *Ocimum sanctum, Cinnamomum zeylanicum, Xanthoxylum armatum and Origanum majorana*. *Kathmandu University Journal of Science, Engineering And Technology*. 2009;5(1):pp 143- 50.

STUDY OF THE ANTIBACTERIAL EFFECT OF MANY PLANTS ON *PSEUDOMONAS AERUGINOSA* WHICH REVEAL RESISTANT AGANIST MANY ANTIBIOTICS

ABSTRACT

Background: Pathogenic germs have developed an increasing resistance toward many antibiotics which form a true problem to human being, because these germs can pass to humans through several substance such as water, food and air that may cause many dangerous diseases.

Object: The aim of this study is to investigate the effect of extractions prepared from different parts of the flowing plants: *Olea europea Linn (Oleaceae)*, *Myrtus communis Linn (Liliaceae), Majorana syriacus Linn (Laminaceae)*, Zingiber officinale *Linn (Zingiberaceae),* and *Achillea falcata Linn (Asteraceae),* against *Pseudomonas Aeruginosa.*

Materials and methods: We performed this work in four stages: First of all, we investigated the presence of *Pseudomonas Aeruginosa* in 667 Samples of milk by using blood agar, selective agar for growing *Pseudomonas Aeruginosa, and* Analytical Profile Index(API20e). Secondly, we extracted the previous plants with water, absolute alcohol, then ether by using soxhlet apparatus and rotary vacuum evaporator. Thirdly, we determined the antibacterial activity of many antibiotics by using disc diffusion method (Muller-Hinton agar). Fourthly, we determined the antibacterial activity of the extractions by using disc diffusion method.

Results: This study has shown the presence of different antibacterial effect of the extracts prepared from different parts of these plants. The extraction of *Achillea falcata* has the strongest effect against *Pseudomonas Aeruginosa* whereas the extraction of Zingiber officinale has the weakest effect against *Pseudomonas Aeruginosa.* The studied antibiotics did not show any antibacterial effect against these germs except Amikacin which has an acceptable effect against those germs.

Conclusion: Since the alcoholic extractions of the studied plants have an antibacterial effect, we recommend to investigate the probable antibacterial effect of those plants against other germs specially that have shown resistance toward antibiotics.

Keywords: Olea europea, Achillea falcate, Majorana syriacus, Pseudomonas Aeruginosa

INTRODUCTION

Researchers have been trying to develop new broad-spectrum antibiotics to stand against infectious diseases .Prolonged usage of these broad-spectrum antibiotics has led to the emergence of drug resistance. That directed the researcher to medical plants. Therefore we tried in our research to investigate the possibility to plants with the capacity to confront empower bacteria. The extracts of *Olea europea Linn (Oleaceae)*, *Myrtus communis Linn (Liliaceae), Majorana syriacus Linn (Laminaceae)*, were prepared from leaves, flowers of *Achillea falcate* (Asteraceae), *and roots of* Zingiber officinale *Linn (Zingiberaceae).*

The Olea europea *Linn* from the Oleaceae, is an evergreen long-lasting fruit tree, and is rooted in the Mediterranean region [1]. It is worth mentioning that many studies have proven its antimicrobial activity [2-4].

Myrtus communis *Linn* back to the Liliaceae, is an evergreen, bushy shrub or a small tree growing up to 5 m high with opposite branches. The dark green leaves are glossy, glabrous, coriaceous, opposite-paired or whorled, ovate to lanceolate, entire-margined, acuminate [5]. Many studies have shown its antibacterial effect [6, 7].

Majorana syriacus *Linn (Marjoram or Origanum syriaca L.)* (Laminaceae family). The genus Origanum majorana L. is an aromatic, perennial, herbaceous plant. The plant has been used as a flavouring and herbal spice from time immemorial. The plant is pungent, bitter, hot, stomachic, anthelmintic, alexipharmic, useful in diseases of the heart and blood, fevers, leucoderma and inflammation. The plant is reported to posse antibacterial activity [8].

Zingiber officinale *Linn (Zingiberaceae)*, is a minor chemical irritant, and has a sialagogue action. Mature *Zingiber officinale (Ginger)* roots are fibrous and nearly dry. Its roots are used as spice in cooking [9]. *Ginger* possesses other interesting pharmacological and physiological properties. For instance, it acts as an anti-inflammatory, analgesic, antipyretic, anti-hepatotoxic and cardiotonic substance. Several studies also revealed its anti-bacterial effect [10, 11]. The main constituents of Ginger are sesquiterpenoids with zingiberene as the main component. Gingerone, shoagoles and gingerols, volatile oils [9]. Gingerol-related components have been reported to possess antimicrobial and antifungal properties, as well as several pharmaceutical properties [12].

Finally Achillea falcata Linn backs to the Asteraceae, is a herb perennial, ranging in height from 20 to 70 cm and sometimes higher. The stem coated hairs has aromatic odor. The leaves are light green, small, long, and gear .The flowers have yellow color, which grows in the Badia region of Syria. Some studies have proved to its anti-bacterial effect [13].

Pseudomonas aeruginosa is a sporadic and opportunistic pathogen that is widely distributed in the environment. Significant isolations of this species from skin, ear, mammary and lung infections have been reported .Water can act as an important medium for the spread of *Pseudomonas* infections, particularly in cases of mastitis, rhinitis and otitis. *P. aeruginosa* is considered a cause of nasomaxillary and mandibular osteomyelitis in sheep [14]. It can also invade fertile eggs causing death of embryos and virulent strains can cause diarrhea, dehydration, dyspnea, septicemia and death to newly hatched chicks [15]. As for human *Pseudomonas aeruginosa* is an opportunistic pathogen that causes severe and life-threatening infections in immune-compromised patients such as these with respiratory diseases, burns, cancers undergoing chemotherapy and cystic fibrosis. [16].

THE OBJECT

The search for therapeutic alternatives against these bacteria, especially those resistant to antibiotics, and to select the plant extract which has the strongest antimicrobial effect on these bacteria. This is an important matter for human on many levels. Since microorganisms have developed resistance to many antibiotics, and this has created immense clinical problem in the treatment of infectious diseases. The new in this research is studying the effect of *Majorana syriacus, and Achillea falcate* extracts against *Pseudomonas aeruginosa.*

PLACE AND TIME OF THE STUDY

The study had been conducted from January 2010 through April 2011. The plant extracts were prepared at the laboratories of Agriculture and Pharmacy Faculties - Damascus University.

The bacterial tests were carried out in the veterinarian Central laboratory of Damascus.

MATERIALS

1. Materials and Equipment Necessary to Identify the Bacteria

Oxidase test tablets, *Hydrogen Peroxide* for Catalase test, Kovac Reagent for Indole Test, Blood Agar cultured supplemented with 5% sheep blood without fibrin, an agar cultured special for *Pseudomonas aeruginosa* Isolation agar (HiMedia-India company). All isolates identified by cultural, morphological and biochemical tests. The biochemical tests were:

API20E system (Analytical Profile Index) manufactured by Bio Merieux, France, was performed, that test 23 differential biochemical tests:

- Investigate the effect of enzymes: 2 - nitrophenyl-βD-galactopyranoside, Arginine dihydrolase, oxidase.
- Decarboxylation Interactions of amino acids: L-lysine, L-omithine.
- Deaminase interaction of the amino acid: L-tryptophan.
- Fermentation reactions of the following sugars: D-glucose, D-mannitol, Inositol, D-sorbitol, L-rhamnose, D-sucrose, D-melibiose, Amygdaline Arabinose.
- Production reactions: indole, Asitoen.
- Reactions produce gases: hydrogen sulphide, nitrogen, nitrogen oxide.
- Study the interactions of Recipes: gelatin diluted, citrate use, hydrolysis of urea (urease).

2. Materials and Equipment Required for the Preparation of Plant Extracts

Olea europea, Myrtus communis,and Majorana syriacus leaves, Zingiber officinale roots, and *Achillea falcata* flowers , soxhlet apparatus, rotary vacuum evaporator , lyophilizer.

3. Materials Required for Susceptibility Test

Muller-Hinton agar medium, susceptibility test discs, 0.45 micrometers diameter membrane filters (whatman, UK) [17], standard discs contain certain concentrations of many antibiotics (Bioanalyse).

METHODS

1. Preparing Plant Extracts

Olea, Myrtus, Majorana leaves, and *Achillea* flowers were Collected on the early morning hours during the period from June to August from Damascus rural area, while the Zingiber roots were purchased from Damascus markets, which were identified by Prof. Dr. Anwar Al-Khatib from Damauscs university. The plant were washed with cold water, distilled water, then dried with hot air at a temperature not exceeding 60°C in the shadow. Then were crushed properly by metal mortar until a fine homogeneous powder was obtained, kept in paper bags with free humidity conditions, ready to prepare extract [18].

Plant parts were extracted separately by continuous extraction device (Soxhlet apparatus), adopted method described by Wang [19] for preparing plant extracts by organic solvents. Three different polar solvents have been selected to extract the components of the plants, which are respectively: water, absolute ethanol, and then Light Petroleum. 50 g of plant powder were placed for 4 hours, by an electric mortar, inside the thimble-holder of Soxhlet apparatus, with 500 ml of each organic solvent (rate: 10.1 weight: volume). The ethanol, and potrelium ether extracts were dried using rotary vaccum evaporator at a temperature not exceeding 40°C, while the aqueous extract was dried using lyophilizer, stored in sterile bottles at 4°C for further experiments.

2. Sampling Method

667 milk samples were collected from dairy cows with clinical mastitis (as veterinary diagnosis). The samples were placed in sterile tubes and fitted with a strap closure, and card number includes name of the sample, place, and date of collection. The samples were transported to the laboratory refrigerated (2-4°C) at full speed.

These samples were investigated for the presence of *Pseudomonas aeruginosa*. The bacteria were identified culturally, morphologically and biochemically. Microscopic examination was conducted after 24 hours of incubation on blood agar (HiMedia) plates. All of the following tests were conducted: oxidase, catalase, Indole test.

3. Cultured Method of Pathological Sample

The following information were Registered on the bottom of the Petri-dishes: the number, name of the sample, place, and date of collection. Then the sample was taken by sterile écouvillon, and placed on blood agar (HiMedia) plates, and incubated for 24 hours at 37°C. It is worth mentioning that all the samples were planted within two hours from the time of sampling.

4. Identifying the Bacteria

The bacteria were identified culturally, morphologically and bio-chemically. The API20E system was also used to support the identification process.

Pseudomonas aeruginosa were selected after the following steps:

4.1. Microscopic Examination

Microscopic examination was conducted after 24 hours of incubation on blood agar using the gram stain, and hanging drop method (motility).

4.2. Microbial Selective Cultures

The selective media according to the method of Al-Rifai [20], where the bacteria from blood agar was cultured, then incubated for 20 to 24 hours at 35-37°C.

4.3. Biochemical Tests

All of the following tests were Conducted: oxidase, catalase, indole.

4.4. Analytical Profile Index Technique (API20e)

This technique was performed according to the manufacturer's instructions:

Bacterial colonies were suspended in 0.85% sterile saline to achieve a homogeneous bacterial suspension. The honey-combed of the incubation box were filled with distilled water. The bacterial suspension was distributed into the tubes of the strip (some were completely filled, and some were partially filled, while while to the rest tube a paraffin oil was added), then were incubated for 24 hours at 37°C, after that the appropriate reagents were added. The result was recorded on the result sheet presented by the manufacturer.

5. Antimicrobial Susceptibility

The isolates were individually tested against 18 antibiotics. The results were determined by the disk diffusion method (Becton Dikinson, Microbiology Systems, MD, USA) as described by National Committee For Clinical Laboratory Standards (NCCLS2000) [21].

The tested antibiotics and concentration ranges were as follows: amikacin (30 µg), ampicillin (10 µg), Cephalexin (30 µg), cephalothin(30 µg), Doxycyclin(30 µg), Cefadroxil (30 µg), ciprofloxacin (5 µg), clindamycin (2 µg), chloramphenicol (30 µg), erythromycin (15 µg), gentamicin (10 µg), Norfloxacin (10 µg), Oxytetracycline (30 µg), Pefloxacin (5 µg), Oxacillin (1 µg), Enrofloxacin (5 µg), tetracycline (30 µg) and Amoxicillin(25 µg). The resistance breakpoints were those defined by the National Committee for Clinical Laboratory Standards (NCCLS, 2000) for Gram-negative bacteria [21].

6. A Bacterial Growth Inhibition Test of Plant Extracts by the Disk Diffusion Method

Sterile filter paper disks were impregnated with 5 microliters of the diluted extracts 66 mg /ml (the disk concentration was 0.33 mg / tablet) in ethanol, water, and petroleum ether. All extracts were filter-sterilized using a 0.45 µm membrane filters (whatman, Co., UK). Control disks also prepared with absolute ethanol, Water, and petroleum ether. The Disks were placed in petri dishes containing Mueller Hinton agar and incubated for 17 hours at 37°C. The diameters of the inhibition zones were measured in millimeters, and compared with Control disks, and standard susceptibility disks [22].

RESULTS

1. Identification of the Bacteria

Bacteria samples that gave us the following results were selected:

1.1. Microscopy

Gram-negative bacilli, straight rods with round edges, compatible with reference [20, 23].

1.2. Germ Culture

On blood agar large colonies with irregular edges, induced β-hemolysis, and aromatic odor similar to the smell of apricot blossom. These results is depended according to Al-Rifai, and Ebeid [20, 23].

On *Pseudomonas aeruginosa* isolation agar gray colonies grew. This result is consistent with the appendix of the manufacturer.

1.3. The Results of Biochemical Tests

Oxidase positive: the appearance of purple color [20], catalase positive: bubbles emergence [20], indol negative: no rose ring was observed compatible with reference [20, 23].

1.4. The Results of Analytical Profile Index Technique (API20e)

The results were read after the end of the incubation period, according to the method of manual accompanying the test. The result of reading was: 2216000, which applies to *Pseudomonas aeruginosa* bacteria.

So 89 (13.35%) out of total number 667 samples were obtained from *Pseudomonas aeruginosa.*

Table 1. Diameters of bacterial growth inhibition zones using antibiotics

Antibiotics	diameters zones of inhibition (mm)	Antimicrobial susceptibility results
Oxytetracycline (T)	8-6	Resistant
Amoxicillin(AX)	9-6	Resistant
Oxacillin(OX)	10-7	Resistant
Cefadroxil(CER)	8-6	Resistant
Pefloxacin(PEF)	9 -7	Resistant
Amikacin(AK)	21-19	Sensitive
Tetracyclin(TE)	7-5	Resistant
Ciprofloxacin(CIP)	10 -7	Resistant
Norfloxacin(NOR)	8-5	Resistant
Gentamycin(CN)	8-6	Resistant
Chloramphenicol(C)	8-6	Resistant

Antibiotics	diameters zones of inhibition (mm)	Antimicrobial susceptibility results
Enrofloxacin(ENR)	9 -7	Resistant
Doxycyclin(DO)	9-6	Resistant
Cephalexin(CL)	9-6	Resistant
Cephalotin(KF)	7-5	Resistant
Clindamycin(DA)	9-7	Resistant
Ampicillin(AM)	8-6	Resistant
Erythromycin(E)	9-5	Resistant

2. Antimicrobial Susceptibility Results against Pseudomonas Aeruginosa

Pseudomonas aeruginosa were found resistant to the studied antibiotics, except for amikacin. The diameter of inhibition zones were measured, based on NCCLS 2000 criteria [21], and the standard leaflet of antibiotic discs provided by the manufacturer and the result was 19-21 mm.

3. The Results of Antibacterial Efficacy of Plant Extracts:

The ethanol extracts showed the antibacterial effect, on the contrary, the water and ether petroleum extracts have no antibacterial effect.

Table (2) shows the results obtained of the antibacterial effect for the various extracts obtained from the studied plants, via determination of the diameter zones of inhibition.

Table 2. Antibacterial effect of ethanol extracts of studied plants against Pseudomonas aeruginosa bacteria

Plant	Inhibition zones of Ethanol extracts (mm)
Control/5 μm	0
Achillea falcata flowers	21-24
Myrtus communis leaves	13-17
Olea Europea leaves	10-13
Majorana syriacus leaves	8-10
Zingiber officinale roots	6-9

THE RESULTS OF THE STATISTICAL ANALYSIS

The results were shown in Tables (3-7).

Table 3. Amikacin susceptibility results against Pseudomonas aeruginosa

Classes	x_i	f_i	$f_i . x_i$	$(\mu - x_i)^2$	$f_i (\mu - x_i)^2$
- 19	19.5	35	682.5	$(0.61)^2$	13.02
20- 21	20.5	54	1107	$(-0.39)^2$	8.21
Total		89	1798.5		21.23
Mean $\mu = 20.11$			Stander Division $\sigma = 0.49$		

Table 4. Antibacterial activity of Achillea falcata flowers ethanol extract against Pseudomonas aeruginosa

Classes	x_i	f_i	$f_i . x_i$	$(\mu - x_i)^2$	$f_i (\mu - x_i)^2$
21 -	21.5	18	387	$(1.12)^2$	22.58
22 -	22.5	42	945	$(0.12)^2$	0.60
23 - 24	23.5	29	681.5	$(-0.88)^2$	22.46
Total		89	2013.5		45.64
Mean $\mu = 22.62$			Stander Division $\sigma = 0.72$		

Table 5. Antibacterial activity of *Olea Europea leaves* ethanol extract against Pseudomonas aeruginosa

Classes	x_i	f_i	$f_i . x_i$	$(\mu - x_i)^2$	$f_i (\mu - x_i)^2$
10 -	10.5	17	178.5	$(1.17)^2$	23.27
11 -	11.5	40	460	$(0.17)^2$	1.16
12 - 13	12.5	32	400	$(-0.83)^2$	22.04
Total		274	1038.5		46.47
Mean $\mu = 11.67$			Stander Division $\sigma = 0.72$		

Table 6. Antibacterial activity of *Myrtus communis leaves* ethanol extract against Pseudomonas aeruginosa

Classes	x_i	f_i	$f_i.x_i$	$(\mu - x_i)^2$	$f_i(\mu - x_i)^2$
- 13	13.5	12	162	$(1.80)^2$	38.88
- 14	14.5	20	290	$(0.80)^2$	12.80
- 15	15.5	31	480.5	$(-0.20)^2$	1.24
16 - 17	16.5	26	429	$(-1.20)^2$	37.44
Total		89	1361.5		90.36
Mean $\mu = 15.30$			Stander Division $\sigma = 1$		

Table 7. Antibacterial activity of Zingiber officinale roots ethanol extract against Pseudomonas aeruginosa

Classes	x_i	f_i	$f_i.x_i$	$(\mu - x_i)^2$	$f_i(\mu - x_i)^2$
6 -	6.5	21	136.5	$(1.12)^2$	26.34
7 -	7.5	36	270	$(0.12)^2$	0.52
8 - 9	8.5	32	272	$(-0.88)^2$	24.78
Total		89	678.5		51.64
Mean $\mu = 7.62$			Stander Division $\sigma = 0.76$		

Table 8. Antibacterial activity of Majorana syriacus leaves ethanol extract against Pseudomonas aeruginosa

Classes	x_i	f_i	$f_i.x_i$	$(\mu - x_i)^2$	$f_i(\mu - x_i)^2$
- 8	8.5	41	348.5	$(0.54)^2$	11.96
9- 10	9.5	48	456	$(-0.46)^2$	10.16
Total		89	804.5		22.12
Mean $\mu = 9.04$			Stander Division $\sigma = 0.50$		

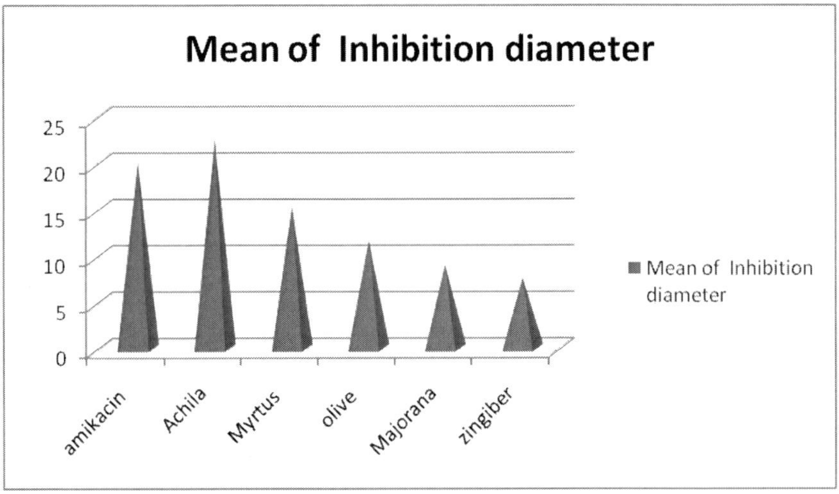

Figure 1. Mean of inhibition diameter of ethanol plants extract and Amikacin against Pseudomonas aeruginosa.

DISCUSSION

The study showed that the percentage of *Pseudomonas aeruginosa* bacteria was (89/667, 13.12%), and this agrees with the study conducted in Korea on contaminated milk samples where it was (20%) [18], and in the Egyptian study too [24].

Pseudomonas Aeruginosa bacteria was resistant to all studied antibiotics except amikacin. As is shown in table (1), that the inhibition diameters of these antibiotics were less than the diameters of bacterial growth inhibition zones adopted in the standards NCCLS2000 [21], and this is consistent with the Korean study where the *Pseudomonas aeruginosa* revealed the highest level of resistance 86.6% [25]. As well as Swartz study, where P. aeruginosa strains, were extremely resistant to all antibiotics tested [26]. But contrarily amikacin showed no bacterial growth in diameter ranged from 19 to 21 mm. So *Pseudomonas Aeruginosa* were sensitive to amikacin, according to the standards NCCLS2000, where the diameter of non-bacterial growth was greater than 14 mm [21]. *Pseudomonas Aeruginosa* showed high resistance to amoxycillin and tobramycin. However, these isolated strains varied in their sensitivity to amikacin, gentamicin, ciprofloxacin, ofloxacin, and cefoperazone [27].

In korean study, amikacin, gentamicin, and piperacillin exhibited strong antimicrobial activities against *Pseudomonas Aeruginosa*, whereas rifampin, cephalothin, cefazolin, and ampicillin were ineffective [25].

The present study demonstrates that ethanolic extract, nor aqueous nither ether petroleum extracts exhibits an inhibitory effect on *Pseudomonas Aeruginosa* growth.

This result comply with the study on bacterial growth inhibition activity of Ginger extracts (n hexane, ethyl acetate, ethanol and water) against several bacteria, which showed that all the extracts except the water extract have antibacterial activity [18].

The results showed variation in the antimicrobial properties of plant extracts (Table 2). The ethanolic extracts showed strong activity (inhibition zone 24 mm), and weak inhibition (zone 6-9 mm). According to this, the major effect was achieved by the ethanolic extracts from *Achillea falcata* flowers, then *Myrtus communis* leaves, followed by *Olea Europea* and *Majorana syriacus* leaves, and the less effect was Zingiber officinale roots extaract.

Comparing the diameter growth inhibition by alcoholic plant extracts with the diameter non-bacterial growth for amikacin (19 to 21 mm), the *Achillea falcata* flowers extract has the strongest effect in inhibiting the growth of *Pseudomonas aeruginosa*, where the diameter of growth inhibition was 24-21 mm. This is compatible with many studies that showed antibacterial effect by several extracts of different types of *Achillea* flowers aganist many bacteria including *Pseudomonas* [13, 14].

The antibacteria effect of the ethanol extract of *Myrtus communis* leaves was revealed in inhibition diameters ranged from 13 to 17 mm. That complys with the powerful antibacterial effect by the ethanol extract against a range of food-borne pathogens and food spoilage bacteria. on food contaminated [16]. The study was endorsed by the Iranian group of plants that have demonstrated the effect of essential oils of *Myrtus communis* leaf against *Pseudomonas aeruginosa* strain [18].

Olive leaf has exhibited non-bacterial growth diameter ranged from 10 to 13 mm. Many studies showed antibacterial effect of olive leaf [2, 26]. Some researchers have demonstrated that biocompounds present in olive products, such as oleuropein and hydroxytyrosol and aliphatic aldehydes, inhibit the growth of a range of bacteria and microfungi [24, 27]. The antibacterial effect of Oleuropein by damaging the bacterial membrane and/or disrupting cell peptidoglycans [27].

The diameter inhibition of growth by *Majorana syriacus* leaves ranged from 8 to 10 mm. An Indian's study confirmed the antibiotics effect of the *Origanum majorana L.* aganist *Pseudomonas aeruginosa* [8].

Ginger (Zingiber officinale Roscoe) and its gingerol-related components have been reported to possess antimicrobial and antifungal properties, as well as several pharmaceutical properties [12]. As well as Malu study showed that Ginger extracts (n-hexane, ethyl acetate, ethanolic soxhlet) except the water extract have antibacterial activity [28).Which comply with our results.

Conclusion

The results showed variation in the antimicrobial properties of ethanol plant extracts. The major effect was achieved by the ethanol extracts from *Achillea falcata* flowers, then *Myrtus communis* leaves, followed by *Olea Europea* and *Majorana syriacus* leaves, and the less effect was Zingiber officinale roots extaract.

References

[1] Belaj, A; Satovic, Z; Rallo, L; Trujillo, I. Genetic diversity and relationships in olive (Olea europaea L.) germplasm collections as determined by randomly amplified polymorphic DNA. *TAG Theoretical and Applied Genetics*. 2002;105(4):638-44.

[2] Bisignano, G; Tomaino, A; Cascio, RL; Crisafi, G; Uccella, N; Saija A. On the in-vitro antimicrobial activity of oleuropein and hydroxytyrosol. *Journal of pharmacy and pharmacology*. 1999;51(8):971-4.

[3] Markin, D; Duek, L; Berdicevsky, I. In vitro antimicrobial activity of olive leaves. *Mycoses*. 2003;46(3-4):132-6.

[4] Pereira, AP; Ferreira, IC; Marcelino, F; Valentão, P; Andrade, PB; Seabra, R; et al. Phenolic compounds and antimicrobial activity of olive (Olea europaea L. Cv. Cobrançosa) leaves. *Molecules*. 2007;12(5):1153-62.

[5] Gruenwald, J; Brendler, T; Jaenicke, C. Physicians' Desk Reference (PDR) For Herbal Medicines: Medical Economics Company; 2000.

[6] Khder, AK. Effect of Allium sativum and Myrtus communis on the elimination of antibiotic resistance and swarming of Proteus mirabilis. *Jordan Journal of Biological Sciences (JJBS)*. 2008:3124.
[7] Al-Anbori, DK; Al-Nimer, MS; Al-Weheb, AM. Athraa M:Antibacterial activity of ethanolic extract of Myrtus communis. L leaves against salivary Mutans streptococci. *Saudi Dental Journal*. 2008;20(3):82-7.
[8] Leeja, L; Thoppil, J. Antimicrobial activity of methanol extract of Origanum majorana L.(Sweet marjoram). *Journal of Environmental Biology*. 2007;28(1):145.
[9] Marks, SL; Kather, EJ. Antimicrobial susceptibilities of canine Clostridium difficile and Clostridium perfringens isolates to commonly utilized antimicrobial drugs. *Veterinary microbiology*. 2003;94(1):39-45.
[10] Philip, K; Malek , SNA; Sani, W; Shin, SK; Kumar, S; Lai, HS; et al. Antimicrobial activity of some medicinal plants from Malaysia. *American Journal of Applied Sciences*. 2009;6(8):1613-7.
[11] Akoachere, J; Ndip, R; Chenwi, E; Ndip, L; Njock, T; Anong, D. Antibacterial effects of Zingiber Officinale and Garcinia Kola on respiratory tract pathogens. *East African medical journal*. 2006;79(11):588-92.
[12] Park, M; Bae, J; Lee, DS. Antibacterial activity of [10]-gingerol and [12]-gingerol isolated from ginger rhizome against periodontal bacteria. *Phytotherapy Research*. 2008;22(11):1446-9.
[13] Karaalp, C; Yurtman, AN; Karabay; Yavasoglu, NU. Evaluation of antimicrobial properties of Achillea L. flower head extracts. *Pharmaceutical biology*. 2009;47(1):86-91.
[14] Khalil, A; Dababneh, BF; Al-Gabbiesh, AH. Antimicrobial activity against pathogenic microorganisms by extracts from herbal Jordanian plants. *Journal of Food, Agriculture & Environment*. 2009;7(2):103-6.
[15] Aburjai, T; Hudaib, M. Antiplatelet, antibacterial and antifungal activities of Achillea falcata extracts and evaluation of volatile oil composition. *Pharmacognosy Magazine*. 2006;2(7):191.
[16] Amensour, M; Bouhdid, S; Fernandez-Lopez, J; Idaomar, M; Senhaji, NS; Abrini, J. Antibacterial activity of extracts of Myrtus communis against food-borne pathogenic and spoilage bacteria. *International Journal of Food Properties*. 2010;13(6):1215-24.
[17] Radulović, N; Stankov-Jovanović, V; Stojanović, G; Šmelcerović, A; Spiteller, M; Asakawa,Y. Screening of in vitro antimicrobial and antioxidant activity of nine Hypericum species from the Balkans. *Food chemistry*. 2007;103(1):15-21.

[18] Owlia, P; Saderi, H; Rasooli, I; Sefidkon, F. Antimicrobial characteristics of some herbal Oils on Pseudomonas aeruginosa with special reference to their chemical compositions. *Iranian Journal of Pharmaceutical Research.* 2010;8(2):107-14.

[19] Wang, L; Weller, CL. Recent advances in extraction of nutraceuticals from plants. *Trends in Food Science & Technology*. 2006;17(6):300-12.

[20] Al-Rifai, I; Alomar, A. special Microbiology 2007:106-7.

[21] Wilker, MA; Cockerill, FR; Craig, WA; Dudley, MN; Eliopoulos, GM; Hecht, DW. M100-S17 Performance Standards for Antimicrobial Susceptibility Testing; Seventeenth Informationl Supplement. 2007;27(1).

[22] Pradeep, B; Manojbabu, M; Palaniswamy, M. Antibacterial Activity of Punica granatum L. Against Gastro Intestinal Tract Infection Causing Organisms. *Ethnobotanical Leaflets*. 2008;2008(1):143.

[23] Ebeid, M. microbiology. 4th ed: Publications of the University of Damascus; 2000.

[24] Tafesh, A; Najami, N; Jadoun, J; Halahlih, F; Riepl, H; Azaizeh, H. Synergistic antibacterial effects of polyphenolic compounds from olive mill wastewater. *Evidence-Based Complementary and Alternative Medicine*. 2011;2011.

[25] Nam, H; Lim, SK; Kang, HM; Kim, JM; Moon, JS; Jang, KC; et al. Antimicrobial resistance of streptococci isolated from mastitic bovine milk samples in Korea. *Journal of Veterinary Diagnostic Investigation*. 2009;21(5):698.

[26] Sudjana, AN; D'Orazio, C; Ryan, V; Rasool, N; Ng, J; Islam, N; et al. Antimicrobial activity of commercial Olea europaea (olive) leaf extract. *International journal of antimicrobial agents*. 2009;33(5):461-3.

[27] Omar, SH. Oleuropein in olive and its pharmacological effects. *Scientia pharmaceutica*. 2010;78(2):133.

[28] Malu, S; Obochi, G; Tawo, E; Nyong, B. Antibacterial activity and medicinal properties of ginger (Zingiber officinale). *Global journal of pure and applied sciences*. 2009;15(3):365-8.

INDEX

#

A

B

D

E

F

G

H

I

J

K

L

M

N

Q

R

S

T

U

V

W

Y

Z

α

β